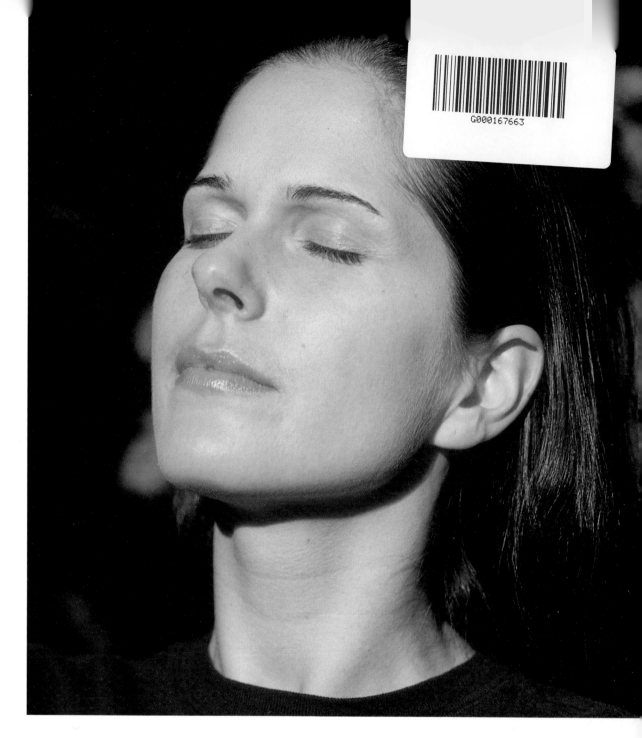

ABOVE

Nearly everyone enjoys the warmth of sunlight on the face, and there is plenty of evidence that sunbathing can make you feel better in yourself. Sunlight also has plenty of physical benefits.

For example, UV rays stimulate the body's calcium and phosphate balance, encourage calcium absorption from the gut, and help keep bones and teeth strong. However, sunlight can also have major downsides. Too much UV light not only burns the

skin but is the major cause of premature ageing of the skin. And, more worrying, it can also cause melanoma skin cancer. So as with so many things in life, getting the right balance – of enough, but not too much – is everything.

what skin needs

There are many simple, practical ways of helping your skin carry out its important tasks. Some involve caring from within, others from without.

SKIN-CARE FROM WITHIN

Your skin's well-being relies on getting the right supply of nutrients, water, oxygen, hormones and neurotransmitters (substances that enable nerve fibres to carry messages) from the blood. However, many things can prevent an adequate supply. Find out how to avoid or correct them, if possible, in Chapters 3–6. They include:

- an unhealthy diet, which reduces the skin's nutrient supply and encourages heart disease due to a narrowing of the arteries with 'bad' cholesterol – there are two basic types of cholesterol: low-density lipoprotein cholesterol (LDL-C) and high-density lipoprotein cholesterol (HDL-C); too much cholesterol, and too much LDL-C compared to HDL-C, along with an unhealthy lifestyle (such as a poor diet, not enough exercise, smoking, and continued over-stress), leads to the laying-down in the arteries of oxidized LDL-C or 'bad' cholesterol in a layer of fatty material called atheroma
- poor digestion, which reduces the skin's nutrient supply
- a low fluid intake, which dehydrates skin cells
- a lack of regular exercise, which encourages heart disease due to the narrowing of the arteries with 'bad' cholesterol and can have adverse effects on the levels of various hormones which are important to the skin, including insulin (which regulates blood sugar and fats) and oestrogen (which helps keep skin cells plump)
- anything that causes fluid retention and hampers the removal of tissue fluid in blood and lymph, so encouraging puffiness, including food sensitivity; pre-menstrual syndrome (PMS); pregnancy; and heart, kidney or liver disease
- being over-stressed, which produces stress hormones that narrow arteries and also encourage the deposition of 'bad' cholesterol
- smoking, which narrows arteries and encourages them to 'fill up' with deposits of 'bad' cholesterol
- an unhealthy breathing pattern, which reduces the oxygen available to skin cells
- heart disease, which reduces blood flow through the skin
- lowered production of certain hormones (the effects depend on the particular hormone) – examples include a lack of thyroxine (making skin dry and cold, and eyebrow and eyelash hairs fall); a lack of oestrogen (making skin thinner and skin cells less plump, and encouraging dry, lined skin); and a lack of insulin (encouraging 'bad' cholesterol to narrow arteries)
- low levels of neurotransmitters, which can prevent good regulation of the blood supply, disturb sebum and sweat production, and trigger a low mood that encourages frowning and drooping of the mouth
- over-sensitivity to temperature changes, which can make arteries suddenly constrict or relax
- poor sleep (either too few hours at a stretch, or broken sleep) – it's during our sleeping hours that we produce the highest levels of the various hormones (including growth hormone) and other factors that encourage skin

the
feel-good
facelift

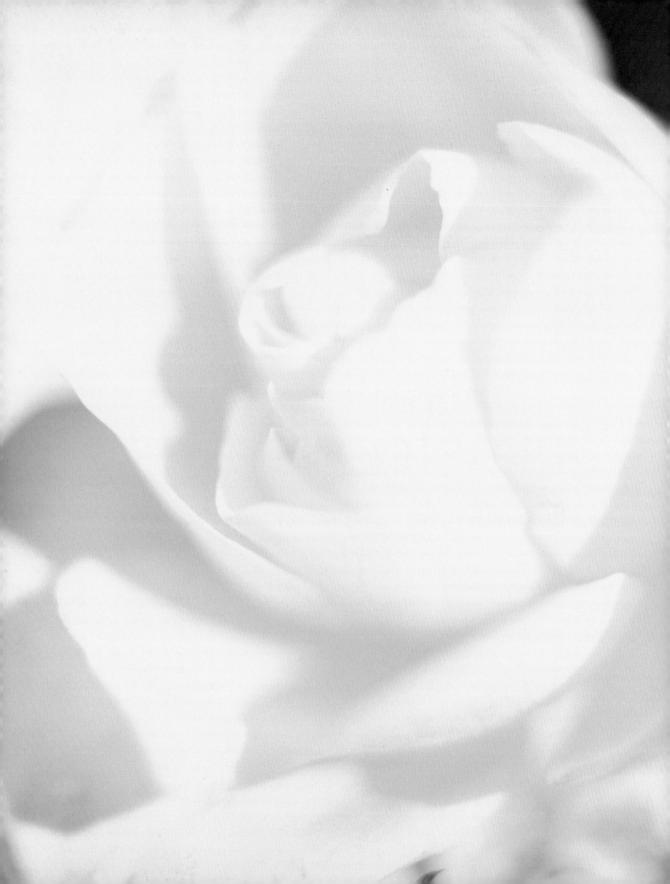

the feel-good facelift

the natural way to look and feel younger

penny stanway

photography by laura hodgson

Kyle Cathie Limited

This book is dedicated to anyone who desires a new shine in their eyes, a new loveliness in their looks and a new feel-good factor in their heart, mind and soul.

acknowledgements

With warm thanks to my editor, Kate Oldfield, her assistants, Sheila Boniface and Andrie Morris, my copy editor, Ruth Baldwin and my proofreader, Tasha Goddard for their expertise, encouragement and enthusiasm; Mark Latter, for creating such a relaxing, 'feel-good' design, Laura Hodgson, for her artist's eye; and the models – Denise Rivett, Sola Abdul and my daughter, Susie Stanway, for allowing their natural beauty to grace and enhance this book.

All photography by Laura Hodgson except for the following: 6 and 35, Michelle Garrett; 23 and 145, Tony Stone Images; 57, The Image Bank/Terje Rakke.

This edition first published in Great Britain, 2000 by

Kyle Cathie Limited

122 Arlington Road London NW1 7HP

ISBN 1 85626 361 4

Text © 2000 Dr Penny Stanway

Photography © 2000 Laura Hodgson

Edited by Kate Oldfield

Production by Lorraine Baird and Sha Huxtable

Copy edited by Ruth Baldwin

Proofreading by TAG

Designed by Vivid

Colour repro: Chroma Graphics

contents

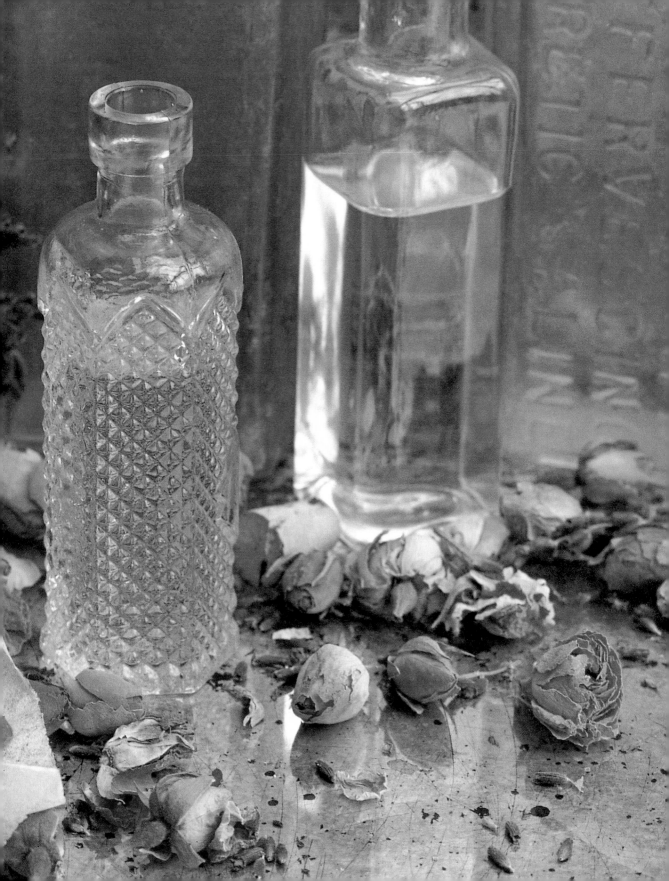

introduction

I have written this book because I'm alarmed by the huge increase in cosmetic surgery and feel strongly that more information should be made available on all the other safe, effective ways of giving the face a lift. Many of these are lovely to use and, as part of a package, may well prolong your life.

WHY A FACELIFT AT ALL?

Many people think about such things as a surgical facelift; a laser or chemical peel; dermabrasion (sandpapering or other mechanical removal of the skin's surface); or injections of botulinum toxin, collagen or fat. And more and more actually have one or more of them done.

A major high-street bank recently revealed that nearly one in five personal loans is taken out to pay for cosmetic surgery. Another recent survey found that one woman in three under the age of forty toys with the idea of having 'aesthetic' plastic surgery – cosmetic surgery to change her looks. Many more over-forties do so. And each year hundreds of thousands of women around the world have cosmetic facial surgery, or some other invasive cosmetic facial procedure.

Precise figures are impossible to obtain because so few private hospitals register how many of these operations they do, let alone how many of each sort they do. However, in the UK, we know that around 65,000 cosmetic operations are done annually – which means an astonishing one in 770 people agrees to have their face or body treated this way in any one year. One expert reckons that around 20 percent of such operations are on the face and eyes. If you include laser resurfacing of the face, the figure

jumps to around 33 percent. So as an estimate, that means between 13,000 and 22,000 people allow their face to go under the knife or laser beam in any one year. (This figure excludes the 7000 or more who have a rhinoplasty, or 'nose job'). Applying the same calculations to the USA, where 2,100,000 people (one in 500 of the population) have cosmetic surgery each year, then between 400,000 and 700,000 have surgery or laser resurfacing of their face in any one year. The percentages are even higher among the monied classes of certain South American countries, such as Brazil. And they are not much lower in other westernized countries, such as Germany, Australia and South Africa.

WHY MOSTLY WOMEN?

Nine out of ten of those who have a surgical or laser 'facelifting' procedure are women. Given that most are over forty, it is clear that age must have something to do with their decision. Either they want to rejuvenate their looks by attempting to reverse certain age-related skin changes, or they or their partners are now in a position to pay for something the woman has wanted for some time. The truth probably lies somewhere between the two, with the wish to counteract ageing being the more important.

what your face reveals

Many people – men and women – in western cultures see the age-related changes of their face as negative and want to look more like they did when younger. Some justifiably fear that such changes mean they are less sexually attractive. Others fear losing their job, or having difficulty in finding one. Many want to look more youthful for their own sake, or because their friends have had a facelift and they want to follow the trend. And for some men and women, image really is everything.

In their quest for youth many people are not much concerned about the potential hazards of surgery. They do not realize there are alternatives. They do not know that surgically induced 'youth' quickly fades.

However, the face reveals the effects of many influences, both internal and external, other than ageing. So having a surgical facelift could be a fool's errand, because if certain conditions continue, its rejuvenating effects will not last. This is why the best cosmetic surgeons always advise on lifestyle changes. Indeed, it could be argued that this advice has many more long-term benefits for their patients' faces than does surgery.

Of course, you can follow this lifestyle advice without having the surgery at all. And you can do very much more besides.

For each individual's face is like a map, in that it records certain aspects of their physical and emotional 'geography'. While our genes dictate the basic structure, our physical, mental and spiritual experiences can powerfully influence the way in which each part of the face works. This, in turn, affects whether it is actually as young as – or old – as it appears.

APPARENT AGE, BIRTH AGE AND PREMATURE AGEING

A person's apparent age – the age they look (sometimes, rather confusingly, called their 'biological' age) – may not equate with their actual chronological or 'birth' age. If the skin, muscles, nerves, blood vessels, lymph vessels and connective tissues of the face are working well, the face looks younger than it would if one or more of these were unhealthy or 'out of sorts'. The converse is equally true. There are three major influences on how each type of tissue works: genetics, 'illness history' and lifestyle.

If an illness or detrimental lifestyle has damaged the way one or more of these tissues in the face works, there may be a discrepancy between the individual's birth age and their apparent age. If the damage is pronounced enough, the person may appear prematurely aged. Examples of factors that can lead to premature ageing include:

- a poor diet and lack of exercise, which cause 'bad' cholesterol (oxidized low-density lipoprotein, see page 20) to be deposited in the arteries, so restricting the blood supply to the skin, muscles and nerves

- repeated, fast, poor-quality slimming diets, which rapidly remove fat from the face and lead to sagging
- stress, which leads to unwanted lines
- smoking, which produces a 'kippered' effect of the facial skin
- lack of sleep, which may decrease keratin and collagen production.

PAST SKIN-CARE AND PROBLEMS

Your skin reveals clues about how you treat it now, and how you treated it in the past. Excessive sun exposure, for example, is the most potent cause of premature ageing of facial skin. Dryness could indicate a poor diet, over-exposure to harsh weather or a low humidity in your home or workplace.

YOUR EMOTIONAL STATE

The face offers the conscious and unconscious mind a powerful way of expressing emotions. (Other ways of doing this include the tone, pitch, timbre and volume of the voice; the content and speed of a person's speech; their posture and gestures; the style, colour and upkeep of their clothing; and their behaviour.) This means your expressions readily reveal your emotional state, unless you consciously strive to keep your feelings hidden. The emotions habitually expressed in the face help shape and contour it in a way that gives each individual a unique appearance. This 'map' is what others know us by and may even love us for.

CHARACTER, FACE READING AND PHRENOLOGY

It's a paradox that our character influences our face, and our face influences our character. The way we think, feel and behave alters the set of our muscles, eyes, mouth and jaw, the lines on our face and the quality of our skin. So this causes permanent structural changes as well as temporary ones. In turn, these changes influence other people's behaviour towards us, which can then affect our personality.

It may be possible to get other clues about a person's character, health and current emotional state from their face. This 'face reading', or physiognomy, is a spin-off from phrenology, the once-popular study of alleged connections between the shape of the various skullbones and the abilities of the underlying parts of the brain.

SPIRITUAL WELL-BEING

Your 'spirit' or 'soul' is a vitally important influence on your looks. Many people find that paying attention to this part of themselves enriches their lives. In turn, a rich and active spiritual life enlivens their face and can give it a serenity and joy that counteracts the effects of such mundane things as sun-damage. For it fosters an acceptance of what life brings, an understanding of where humans fit into the scheme of things, and the habit of looking at everyday stresses and strains as challenges, not problems.

Precise definitions of the words, 'spirit' and 'soul', belong to the semantics of philosophy and theology. But words aside, each person's spirit/soul is of vital concern to them and the way they look. It's the part that lets us transcend our experiences, thoughts, emotions, behaviour and character. It's the part that can connect us at some deep level with every other living thing on the planet. And it's the part that yearns for communication with the creative being that many of us call God.

cosmetic surgery, other 'invasive' therapies and beauty therapy

Look in the back of any women's glossy magazine and you will see more advertisements for cosmetic surgery and other invasive cosmetic procedures than for almost anything else.

Unfortunately, though, all is not what it seems. Some clinics offering such treatments are staffed by doctors who lack sufficient training to be considered by fully trained, experienced cosmetic surgeons as capable of operating without supervision. The fact that they operate on the face makes it even worse, because any lack of expertise shows so readily here. Worse still, some clinics are so eager to make money from unsuspecting clients that they encourage them to have operations or procedures that were not requested and which any normal observer would deem completely unnecessary.

Nonetheless there are many highly reputable cosmetic surgeons and many people are delighted with the results of their work. But you owe it to yourself to check on the specialist qualifications of any doctor who offers to operate on you.

Another rapidly growing area is laser therapy. Various types of laser can, for example, reduce scarring by peeling the skin; be used as a scalpel during a facelift; and remove unwanted hair. Some more of the many cosmetic procedures available are the injection of Botox (botulinum toxin) to iron out frown marks temporarily; and the peeling of the skin with acid or one of many types of mechanical tool.

Before agreeing to any such procedure, ask how many identical procedures the operator has done. Ask how soon the procedure is likely to need redoing. Ask about complication and failure rates. Ask how their insurance cover protects you. And ask about the full cost.

Most important, however, ask yourself whether you know all you need to know about the alternative: a natural facelift.

GIVING YOURSELF A NATURAL FACELIFT

Anyone can give themselves a natural facelift by using a programme of thoughtful skin-care routines, pleasant-to-use home treatments and simple changes to their lifestyle. If you decide to follow this route, then as you continue with the programme over the weeks and months you will gradually notice that:

- your skin becomes brighter and more resilient, perhaps regaining some of its youthful thickness
- any puffiness is reduced
- fine lines look increasingly less apparent
- your facial contours become more rounded as your facial muscle tone improves
- eye bags and circles diminish
- your eyes sparkle more.

All these effects combine to give a 'lift' to your whole face, decreasing some of the effects of ageing, but without removing its essential character. What's more, they are free from side effects or complications and also generally inexpensive. An added bonus of giving yourself a natural facelift is that doing so will make your whole life more pleasant. It will make you more likely to live out your maximum potential lifespan without dying prematurely. And it isn't just your face that will benefit from this life-changing programme.

A NATURAL FORM OF HRT

One other important benefit of a natural facelift concerns women whose levels of oestrogen and progesterone are falling, low or otherwise unbalanced around the menopause. For many of the lifestyle changes that underpin a natural facelift also balance the levels of these (and other) hormones. So in essence by giving yourself a natural, 'feel-good' facelift, you are giving yourself a natural form of hormone replacement therapy (HRT). Balancing your oestrogen and progesterone this way is one reason why your skin will look better and resist – to some extent – the increase in the rate of ageing of the skin that some women experience at this time of life.

DOES HAVING A NATURAL FACELIFT MEAN HAVING BEAUTY THERAPY?

We can all give ourselves a natural facelift as we go about our daily life in the comfort of our own home, or at work, without ever needing expensive and time-consuming help from a professional beauty therapist. However, some parts of the natural facelift programme in

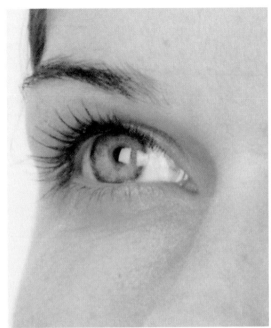

this book are basically types of DIY (do-it-yourself) beauty therapy – treatments aimed at boosting the health of your skin or other parts of your face, and making them look better. And many can, if you wish, involve help from an amateur beauty therapist in the form of a willing friend or family member. But if you want to add sessions of beauty therapy from a professional to your natural facelift programme, all well and good.

WHY A FEEL-GOOD NATURAL FACELIFT?

No facelift other than the natural one described here has such far-reaching benefits. Besides the physical benefits already described, this book will show you how to celebrate your face, become empowered to enjoy your life more and, most important, find an inner radiance. Read on and you will not only see yourself looking your best, but you will also feel better in body, mind and spirit.

part one
tools

The five decades leading up to Y2K – the year 2000 – have seen great leaps forward in two important areas to do with health and beauty maintenance, enhancement and treatment. First, there has been an unprecedented explosion of scientific research in every area; second, there has been an astonishing awakening of interest in the use of complementary and alternative therapies and techniques.

This huge amount of research has led to fascinating advances in our understanding of the things that influence the structures that form our face: our skin, muscles, nerves, blood vessels, connective tissue, bones and hair. And the interest in complementary and alternative healing means we now have ready access to gentle, yet at the same time amazingly powerful ways of helping ourselves and each other look and feel good.

So read on to discover the tools you need to keep you and your face looking and feeling their best. We'll start with updating your skin care and choosing or making skin-care products. We'll progress to how food, exercise, breathing and developing an inner radiance, using a number of professional beauty secrets and treating yourself to a face massage, home electrical treatment and various complementary therapies.

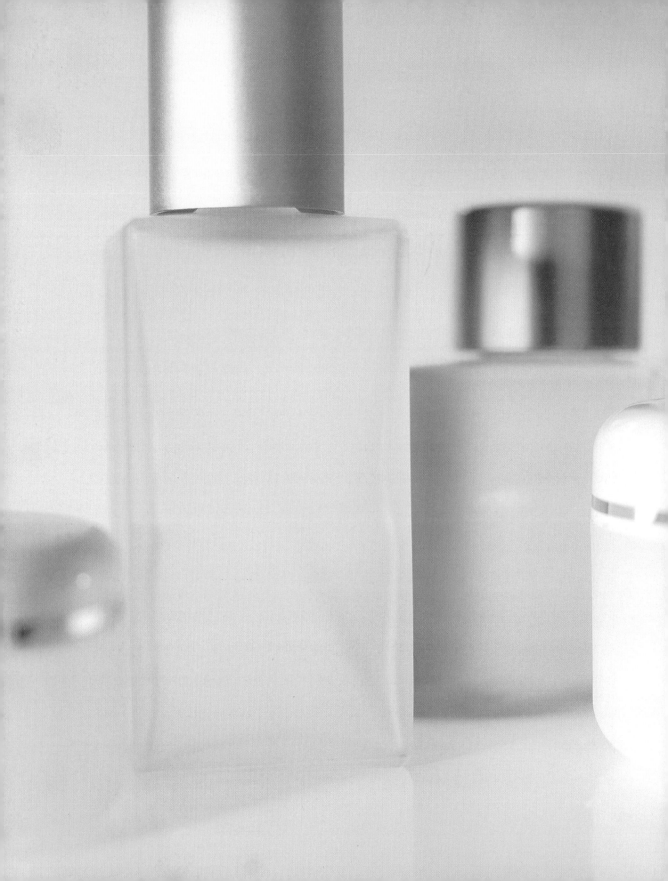

1
updating
your skin-care

Look around any woman's bathroom or bedroom and you'll probably find a large collection of skin-care products, many of them unused, unloved and forgotten. Some will be dry, caked, smelly or past their use-by date, others totally unsuitable. And some, though fresh and new, will be much less effective than others she could have bought – or made herself.

Another undoubtable fact is that some products contain ingredients that are far more active and useful than others. However, you can rarely judge the likely effectiveness of a product by its price. When choosing products, bear in mind the current state of your skin and be aware of which ingredients will best suit your skin. And every so often, have a really good springclean and throw out anything that doesn't deserve a place.

your skin

The skin you see is the surface of the epidermis – the outer layer of skin and the part that forms the roof of a blister. You may think the epidermis is the most important part of the skin because it's what you see. But the dermis forms the bulk of the skin and is also vitally important. The epidermis and dermis are intimately 'glued' together at the layer called the basement membrane, and this prevents them sliding apart.

Most beauty experts advise only on how to look after the epidermis. Of course, using skin-care products can be useful and pleasurable, and make-up can enhance looks and cover uneven colouration. However, if you want to give yourself a natural facelift, you need to boost the well-being of your dermis and basement membrane too. So it's worth becoming acquainted with what goes on in these deeper layers of the skin as well its more superficial part.

NEW SKIN FOR OLD

The outer layer of skin is mainly made of tightly packed keratinocytes, cells that produce keratin, a protein that strengthens the skin and gives it body. These cells produce an oily substance – the skin's own moisturizer – that helps them stick together and, along with sebum (see page 18), helps keep skin supple, waterproof and water-retentive.

The mechanical barrier formed by these keratinocytes helps protect the body from invasion by such things as water, hazardous chemicals, and micro-organisms.

But it's at the base of the epidermis that the most important activity takes place. Here, new keratinocytes are created as each existing one splits into two new ones. One of each pair stays put, ready to split again. The other, however, gradually travels up through the epidermis to the skin's surface. The splitting of one keratinocyte, followed by the journey of one its two new 'daughter' cells to the surface of the skin, normally takes about twenty-eight days in young skin, longer in older skin. The continued creation and journeying of new keratinocytes explains how skin can constantly renew itself and also repair itself from breaks such as cuts, grazes and sores.

On its way to the surface, a keratinocyte's shape changes. From being squarish, it slowly becomes flatter. Before it gets to the top, it dies. This means dead keratinocytes form the surface of the skin you see. If you were to look with a microscope you would see a surface formed of many fine scales. This is perfectly normal. If your skin is dry, you can even see these scales with the naked eye.

As we grow older, our previously tightly packed keratinocytes tend to shrink. The resulting gaps within the skin encourage water loss by evaporation from the skin's surface. This means we have to rely more on natural oils produced by the keratinocytes to make our skin waterproof.

Sprinkled among the upwardly mobile keratinocytes are two other types of cells, known as melanocytes and Langerhans cells.

skin colouring

Melanocytes are cells that give the skin its colour. This is because they contain a brown pigment called melanin. The more melanin in the skin, the darker our skin appears. Most of the melanocytes are in the basal layer of the epidermis, where they normally form one in ten of the cells. A darker-skinned person's melanocytes are more active than those of a fairer-skinned one, and so produce more melanin.

THE 'SUNSHADE EFFECT' OF MELANIN

Melanin protects the other skin cells from over-exposure to sunlight by absorbing ultra-violet (UV) rays. When we expose our skin to sunlight, its rays stimulate the melanocytes to become more active and produce more melanin. However, the melanocytes don't keep this protective pigment to themselves. Instead they 'inject' little granules of it into nearby keratinocytes. These pigment granules group together in the part of each keratinocyte that is nearest the skin surface, making pale skin appear tanned. They do this by aligning themselves between the nucleus of the keratinocyte and the sun's UV rays coming through the skin. So in effect they act as a natural sunshade. We make less melanin as we get older, so using other sun protection becomes even more important.

IMMUNE PROTECTION

More than one in fifty of the cells in the epidermis is a Langerhans cell. This cell is like an octopus in that it has several 'tentacles' that spread out between nearby keratinocytes. These tentacles take samples of any foreign matter entering the skin. The Langerhans cell then travels down through the basement membrane into the dermis

and, from there, enters one of the lymph vessels – tiny channels that drain tissue fluid, as 'lymph', away from the skin. The Langerhans cell continues its journey in the lymph until it reaches one of the lymph nodes (sometimes wrongly called 'glands') along the lymph vessel. Here, specialized cells register the presence of the foreign matter that the Langerhans cell has brought. If necessary, such cells set up an antibody production facility so the body can protect itself against potential damage from future invasion by this foreign matter.

STRENGTH AND SUPPLENESS

The cells in the dermis, the fibrocytes, are more widely spaced than are those of the epidermis. Fibrocytes make fibres of a protein called collagen that helps give skin its strength. The collagen surrounds another protein, elastin, which helps make skin supple and resilient. These collagen-elastin fibres form the material between the fibrocytes. However, collagen and elastin are badly damaged by free radicals (hyperactive oxygen molecules) formed, for example, by sun exposure and smoking. They are also gradually destroyed as we age; in the average forty-year-old, half the elastin present at birth has gone and virtually none of it is replaced. A lack of collagen and elastin encourages lines, wrinkles and thin, sagging skin.

CIRCULATION

All the nutrients and oxygen that skin cells need come from blood vessels in the dermis. The tiniest of these small arteries and veins are called capillaries, and they form a branching network throughout the dermis. The skin's blood supply has many hugely important functions. The arteries and veins help stabilize the temperature in the skin – and the rest of the body – by continually adjusting the blood-flow within. They do this by narrowing, which allows less blood to flow through the skin, or widening, which increases the blood-flow. They are enabled to do this by muscle fibres in their walls either contracting (shortening), which makes the space inside the blood vessels smaller and lets less blood flow through, or relaxing (lengthening), which enlarges the space and lets more blood through. A smaller blood-flow allows less heat to escape from the blood, while a larger flow lets more heat out.

Several things can widen or narrow blood vessels, including the air temperature, body temperature, emotion, stress, certain nutrients, hormones and neurotransmitters (substances that enable messages to pass along nerve fibres), and various abnormal conditions. These can have great significance to your feel-good facelift programme. For not only does the blood-flow through the skin affect temperature control, but it also affects the basic well-being of the skin – and therefore of yourself too.

This is because the blood that flows through the vessels:

- supplies nutrients to skin cells and hair roots

- provides skin cells with oxygen
- removes carbon dioxide and other waste products.

NERVE SUPPLY

The skin's nerve fibres are also situated in the dermis. They carry information about pain, temperature and touch to the spinal cord and brain. They are also responsible for making the tiny muscles that control the size of the blood vessels contract or relax.

VITAMIN D PRODUCTION

UV rays from the sun stimulate the skin to make vitamin D, vital for healthy bones. We normally get much more of this vitamin from our skin than from our food.

SEBUM: A NATURAL WATERPROOFER AND SMOOTHER

The skin's natural 'grease', or sebum, is a blend of oils and other substances produced by the sebaceous glands in the dermis. These glands empty into hair follicles, and the face has a particularly large number of them. Sebum lubricates and waterproofs skin and helps prevent moisture in the skin from evaporating – which keeps keratinocytes well hydrated and therefore plumped up, so smoothing the skin. Sebum production can increase temporarily during stress, before a period and around the menopause. As we grow older we tend to produce less, so our skin becomes drier.

SWEAT GLANDS

The sweat glands lie in the dermis and constantly release sweat into hair follicles; the openings of these follicles are sometimes called 'pores'.

to grow and heal: but growth and healing don't kick in properly until we've been asleep for six hours and we needs two hours more to do the job properly.

SKIN-CARE FROM WITHOUT

When thinking about how to care for your skin from without, the very first thing that will probably spring to mind is what you put on it in the way of creams, lotions and other potions. These include a wide variety of skin-care products such as moisturizers and anti-ageing creams. The second thing you think of will probably be make-up. And the third, sun-protection, in the form of products with an SPF (sun protection factor, see page 24) of 15 or more.

However, there are several other 'external' factors to consider. These include the temperature, cleanliness and moisture level of the surrounding air.

Air temperature

While your skin can readily adjust to varying air temperatures by changing its blood supply and sweat production, it is more comfortable both for our face and for the rest of our body to avoid extremes of temperature.

Clean air

The skin is to some extent self-cleansing, in that sweat and sebum wash dirt away. Its surface layer, along with sebum, also help make it resistant to the entry of dirt. However, it is possible for dirt to become ingrained, especially in dry skin. At worst, certain substances can enter the deeper layers of the skin and set up an allergy. And breathing dirty air can, eventually, damage lungs, so reducing their

capacity to oxygenate the skin's blood supply. So all in all it is better for our skin if we breathe clean air.

Humidity

Air that is too dry encourages evaporation of sweat and of the water in the superficial layers of the skin. Skin that does not produce much sebum is particularly prone to these drying effects. The answer is to humidify the air (see page 63; see also 'Positive ions' on the same) and to help waterproof the skin so as to keep moisture in. You can do this through boosting your sebum production by eating a healthy diet containing plenty of foods rich in essential fats (see pages 45–46), taking daily exercise, learning effective stress management and ensuring that you have enough daily daylight exposure. Another way is to apply moisturizer.

Light

Another hugely important way of caring for the skin from without is to get enough sunlight, but not too much. This is discussed on pages 24–25.

Skin-care products and make-up

You can also give your skin external help with skin-care products and, if you wish, with make-up, see page 90.

The many methods of caring for the skin from without are much more familiar. But the fact is that they are actually much less important. Many beauty advisers, and others who should know better, concentrate only on external skin-care. But clearly, it's better for all of us to aim for skin-care that comes from both without *and* within.

skin variation

The appearance and quality of the skin vary enormously from one person to another. They can also change quite markedly from day to day, and from time to time over any one individual's lifespan.

Several factors account for these differences, including the:

- amount of pigmentation with melanin
- level of sebum production
- degree of dryness
- state of the circulation
- efficiency of lymph drainage
- amount of fine lines and wrinkles
- presence of scars, lumps, moles, freckles and age spots
- degree of hairiness
- degree of elasticity.

A person's genetic blueprint influences all these. However, each is also subject to one or more of several lifestyle factors – including what you eat; how much exercise you take; what sort of air you breathe; whether or not you feel over-stressed; how much you expose your skin to the burning and ageing ultra-violet rays of the sun; and whether you know how to choose and use moisturizers and, if necessary, other skin-care products. So you can often do a lot to alter the state of your skin.just by altering some simple, everyday aspects of the way you live,

BASIC SKIN TYPES

One way of classifying skin is according to its degree of pigmentation. Fair skin contains very little melanin; yellow skin has only slightly more; olive skin has quite a lot; and brown or black skin has most.

Sebum production is sometimes related to skin colour. Heavily pigmented skin tends to produce more sebum. This makes it oilier, more waterproof and better hydrated.

Skin pigmentation and sebum production have important implications for how rapidly skin ages. Skin that is well hydrated is less likely to age prematurely, with the development of fine lines and wrinkles, or by sagging. And skin that is well protected from sunlight by pigment is also less likely to age prematurely, because its melanin absorbs UV light, which helps protect it from photo-ageing – the lines, wrinkles and sagging caused by too much UV.

In contrast, fair-skinned individuals tend to produce less sebum. They have drier, less greasy skin with less melanin. And this means they are more likely to notice early age-related changes in their skin.

From a practical point of view, you need to take particular care of your skin if you are fair-skinned, or if, for some reason, you are going through a time of life when your rate of sebum production is lower than usual, or your skin drier than usual.

Quite a few people, especially in their teens and early twenties, produce more sebum in their T-zone – forehead, nose and below the mouth – while the rest of their skin may be much less oily. This is known as combination skin. The central oiliness is a result of the presence of more sebaceous glands in this area of the face.

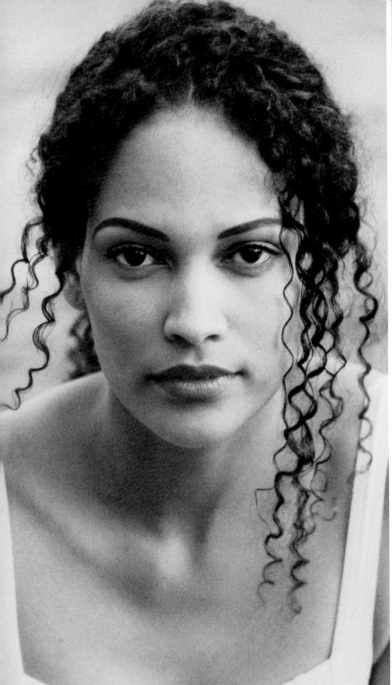

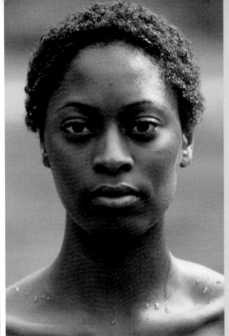

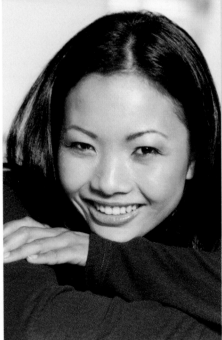

The darker your skin, the more of its 'natural sunshade', melanin, there is in its epidermis, and vice versa. So you'd be right in thinking that paler people burn more readily in the sun. But the fact is that whatever your skin colour, it's perfectly possible for you to become sunburnt from over-exposure to ultra-violet (UV) light. And because too much UV light also ages the skin prematurely and encourages skin cancer, it's clearly wise to know how much sun your skin can take, as well as just how much protection it needs when you're out and about in bright light, especially during the mid-day hours when UV rays are brightest.

Remember that you can burn even on a cloudy day. Go for a product with an SPF (sun protection factor) of 15 and apply it liberally. Researchers say that most people who use a sunscreening product don't put nearly enough on. Reapply it as directed on the packaging, otherwise its effect will wear off.

the sun: friend or foe?

The sun can be a good friend or a bad enemy to the skin. However, a lot of people don't know how best to strike the balance between getting enough sunlight to benefit their skin, yet not so much that it becomes harmful.

The idea that sunlight can be good for us and for our skin (see page 19) is not new. We have known this for years. But too much can cause sunburn and skin cancer. It also results in light-induced ageing (photo-ageing), which is now known to be responsible for 90 percent of premature ageing of the skin. And it thickens the epidermis. Too much sunlight causes these problems partly by creating a large number of hyperactive oxygen particles called free radicals, and partly by encouraging enzymes called metalloproteinases to damage the collagen fibres that provide strength, support and suppleness to the skin.

So while it's certainly wise to enjoy the sun, we should always treat it with great respect.

SUN PROTECTION

Melanin in the skin helps guard against sunburn, photo-ageing and skin cancers (both melanomas and non-melanomas), so the lighter your skin, the higher your risk of sun damage unless you take good care of yourself.

SOLAR UV INDEX

Knowing your risk of burning can be helpful, especially in the summer, when the ultraviolet (UV) rays in sunshine are at their brightest. A guide to your personal risk of burning comes in the form of the daily Solar UV Index, a number from 1 to 20 that is nowadays often given in television weather forecasts and is also available on the Internet. The Solar UV Index is based on the position of the sun in the sky and the amount of cloud cover. Its maximum in the UK is around 8; in southern Europe 10–12; in the southern part of the USA 14–16; and in northern Australia 16–18. Knowing how the Solar UV Index affects your skin type means you know how much sun protection you need.

Protect your skin when necessary with some combination of:

- avoiding the sun, especially between 11am and 3pm
- covering up
- applying liberal amounts of a sunscreening product with a sun protection factor (SPF) of 15 or more – choose a 'reflective' one (such as one containing titanium dioxide; iron or zinc oxide; or magnesium silicate); reapply as directed and, if going swimming, choose a waterproof one or make sure that you reapply sunscreen afterwards
- eating enough foods rich in beta-carotene, vitamins C and E, selenium, zinc and other antioxidants; these nutrients help guard against the production of free radicals – the hyperactive oxygen particles that can damage the skin, but in just half an hour, strong sunlight halves the skin's store of protective vitamin C
- applying plenty of moisturizer after being in sunlight.

SOLAR UV INDEX AND PERSONAL RISK

Skin colour	Solar UV Index								
	1–2	3–4	5	6	7	8	9	10	11–20
White, burns easily, tends not to tan	Low	Med	High	Very high	Very high	Very high	Very high	Very high	High or Very high
White, burns easily	Low	Low	Med	Med	High	High	High	High	High or Very high
Brown	Low	Low	Low	Med	Med	Med	Med	High	High or Very high
Black	Low	Low	Low	Low	Med	Med	Med	Med	High or Very high

Low risk: the sun will not harm you.
Medium risk: do not expose your skin to direct sunlight for more than one to two hours.

High risk: you could burn in thirty to sixty minutes. Try to keep out of direct sunlight, cover up and use a sunscreen of SPF 15 or more.

Very high risk: you could burn severely within twenty to thirty minutes. Stay out of direct sunlight, cover up and use a sunscreen of SPF 15 or more.

If the Solar UV Index is 11 or above, remember that your personal risk level will be either 'high' or 'very high', whatever your skin type.

SUNBEDS

You may like sunbeds, but their UV light can encourage skin cancer. So avoid them if you:

- are under sixteen

- have a history of skin cancer (or have a close relative who has had it)

- suffer from a medical condition that worsens in sunlight

- are on drugs or other remedies that can cause light-sensitivity (such as certain antibiotics, painkillers, antidepressants, 'water tablets', blood-pressure medication, anti-malarial tablets, St John's wort and certain contraceptive pills – check the information in the packet)

- have fair skin that always burns and does not tan – this includes most people with red hair and freckles.

- have lots of moles and/or freckles.

The guidelines for other people are confusing. Many dermatologists believe everyone should avoid sunbeds. The UK's Health and Safety Executive recommends a maximum of twenty sessions a year, as does the Cancer Society of New Zealand. But the European Committee for Electrotechnical Standardization (CENELEC – a committee of trade representatives, scientists and doctors) recommends a limit of sixty a year.

Caution: Always consult a doctor without delay if any mole enlarges, darkens, crusts, bleeds or becomes multi-coloured, irregular or itchy.

skin-care

Advertisements for skin-care products are hugely persuasive and it's always tempting to believe them. We may know a product's ingredients cost only a maximum, on average, of 8 percent of what we paid...

...but many products are delightful to use and most of us thoroughly enjoy opening a new jar of a lightly fragranced, softly coloured, smoothly textured skin-care product, all done up in beautiful wrappings. Simply smoothing on such a product can make you feel a million dollars, quite apart from what it might do to your skin.

Yet these products can be expensive, and their cost may bear little relation to their quality or efficacy. So do we really need them – and, if so, which ones do you personally need?

CLEANSERS

Sebum and sweat production help cleanse skin naturally, and some people with beautiful skin never do anything other than give it an occasional splash with water. Others, however, find their skin is uncomfortably greasy, sticky or smelly at the end of the day, because of the build-up of sebum, sweat and dead skin cells. And those who wear make-up need to remove it every night with a suitable solvent (water for water-based make-up, oil or mild detergent for oil-based make-up). Also, airborne dust, pollens and particles from vehicle-exhaust fumes can become ingrained in the skin's outermost layer, particularly if it's dry and flaky. Such particles can also get trapped in sebum or in the residue from sweat. At worst, dirt blocks hair follicles, encourages pimples and makes the skin look less than its best. This is why many people, especially those living in or near big towns or cities, need some other way of cleaning their skin.

Some choose soap. This can be fine, especially for those with an oily skin. But while it isn't very good at dissolving make-up, it does strip natural and other oils from skin – though the skin replaces its oils within twenty minutes to three hours, depending on its age and condition. Soap also temporarily destroys the skin's natural acidity (though this is also quickly and naturally restored – so don't bother with 'pH balanced' products) and few people are sensitive to perfumes in scented soaps, so always rinse all traces away after washing.

Another option, if you like the feeling of water on your skin, is a soap-free cleansing bar, lotion or cream, but these sometimes make older skin feel tight.

If you use a liquid, cream, gel or foaming cleanser, choose it according to your skin type – cream for dry/mature; lotion for normal; foaming or gel for oily. Massage in thoroughly and remove well afterwards with cotton wool, a soft flannel, or a square of muslin or other light cloth, wrung out in warm water.

TONERS

Toners are often recommended for removing traces of cleanser and the skin's natural oil. They are also said to close 'open pores'. There is no evidence that they are necessary, but if you enjoy the fresh feeling they give, choose an alcohol-free one, unless your skin is very greasy.

MOISTURIZERS

Modern life, with its central heating and air conditioning, readily dehydrates skin, and soap removes natural oils. So many people's skin looks better if they use a moisturizer regularly. And you probably need it if your face still feels tight ten minutes after washing with a cleanser because this suggests that the production of natural oils within your skin is relatively slow. Our natural oil production also varies according to where we are in the menstrual cycle, with more oil being produced in the days leading up to a period. Some slowing of oil production is also natural as we grow older.

A moisturizer adds water to skin and seals in the skin's own moisture; this hydrates keratinocytes and plumps them up for up to twelve hours (which is why you are advised to moisturize twice a day). This can be especially important for older skin, because its fibres of collagen and elastin will be less good at retaining moisture than when they were younger, especially if you're a smoker or your skin shows a lot of photo-ageing. Well-hydrated skin feels comfortable and reflects light so as to look more lustrous.

Choose a moisturizer containing a sunscreen of SPF 15 or more if you are going to be outside for long, or by a sunny window.

Apply your moisturizer to still-moist skin immediately after washing or splashing your face, or using cleanser. The layer of fats that are deposited from the product on to the surface of your skin will then trap a fine layer of extra water next to the skin.

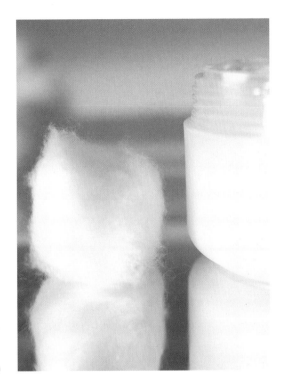

OTHER PRODUCTS

People throughout history have tried to beautify their skin by applying such things as herbal extracts, essential oils, milk, fruit and minerals such as those in clay or mud. Today, skin-care companies put an enormous amount of money and research into finding effective ingredients. Some of these, such as fruit acids (alpha-hydroxy acids), come from age-old skin-care recipes containing fruit or milk; others, such as co-enzyme Q10 (an antioxidant), or stable forms of vitamin A (retinol) and vitamin C, are new.

Certain products are claimed to prevent or reverse lines and wrinkles. However, comparisons of these with ordinary moisturizers suggest that any anti-ageing benefit comes from their moisturizing and sunscreening effects.

which ingredients help and which are over-hyped?

Consumers in many countries can now see what is in a skin-care product from its label, and increasing numbers are taking an interest in exactly what they put on their skin. Some even believe: 'If you can't eat it, don't put it on your skin.'

Strictly speaking, the ingredients in a 'cosmetic' product should not penetrate the dermis, where they could get into blood and lymph and travel around the body, because that would make it a 'medical' product. But skin-care products have always blurred the boundaries between beauty and medicine. In certain circumstances, some ingredients (such as water, alcohol, fats, tiny molecules from essential oils, and petroleum-derived hydrocarbons such as propylene glycol) do enter the dermis, carrying soluble substances with them. However, the amounts that get into blood or lymph are probably too small to have much, if any, effect outside the skin.

Some manufacturers believe they can blind us with science, making extravagant claims for ingredients without explaining what they are, what they are proven to do and whether they do this in the concentrations present in the product. Nonetheless, many products are formulated as a result of much high-tech, high-powered research. And some ingredients do have important properties. Here are just a few of them.

LIPOSOMES AND NANOSPHERES

These minute globular structures deliver substances (that would not get there alone) deep into the epidermis to help plump it up and make it waterproof. There is no comparable equivalent to be used at home.

AHAS

The alpha-hydroxy acids (AHAs) in some commercial skin-care products are natural fruit acids from a variety of foods. Examples are citric, malic, lactic, tartaric, pyruvic and glycolic acids – from lemons, apples, fermented milk, red wine, papaya and sugar cane respectively. These foods have been widely used over the centuries to make home-made beauty products. Alpha-hydroxy acids moisturize skin by attracting water. They may also brighten skin by 'exfoliating' (dislodging dead cells). This makes skin thinner and more prone to sun damage, so be sure to use a sunscreen afterwards.

Alternatively, you can exfoliate dead cells simply by rubbing gently with a towel; benefit from fruit acids in various topically applied foods (applied directly to the skin's surface: see page 40); and use other moisturizers.

VITAMINS

Some studies indicate that applying beta-carotene (the 'pro-vitamin' that our body uses to make vitamin A), vitamin A (retinol), vitamin C and vitamin E directly to the skin helps prevent damage by free radicals – hyperactive oxygen particles which are created by sun exposure, smoking and other physical stresses to the body. Retinol in high enough concentrations acts like tretinoin (see page 131), reducing lines and roughness in photo-damaged skin. It does this by stimulating the production of new skin cells and collagen. Vitamin E also has moisturizing properties; for best results choose a product containing its natural form – d-alpha tocopherol acetate or succinate.

Vitamins A and C are unstable substances, meaning they break down quickly when exposed to air (for example, on the skin), but several products have now been formulated that deliver them intact.

PLANT-DERIVED SUBSTANCES

Certain plant oils and tinctures or extracts have useful effects, and all are available (from certain health-food shops, pharmacies, supermarkets or mail-order suppliers) for making skin-care products at home. Here are some of the most common, along with what they do:

Lavender oil: heals; counteracts infection

Avocado oil: moisturizes; boosts collagen; soothes sunburn; provides vitamin E; lightens

Carrot oil: provides beta-carotene; soothes; counteracts scarring

Jojoba oil (or butter): moisturizes dry skin well; soothes; doesn't go rancid like other oils

Sweet almond oil: provides vitamin E; moisturizes

Wheatgerm oil: softens; soothes; provides vitamin E

Aloe vera gel: soothes sunburn; softens; mild sun-screen; counteracts infection

Butcher's broom extract (Ruscus alculcatus): tightens; lightens

Horsetail extract (Equisetum aruense): tightens

Glycerine: moisturizes

Honey: tightens; counteracts infection

Marigold extract (Calendula officinalis): soothes; softens; freshens

Soya bean extract: tightens

CHOOSING WHAT IS BEST

First, we like skin-care products to look good, smell good and feel good. Second, we want them to do our skin good. You could argue that worrying too much what to choose counteracts the good they do. But before buying a product you might want to consider:

- its price – can you buy (or even make) something similar more cheaply?
- its shelf-life – will you have enough time to enjoy using it before it starts going off
- whether it is organic – some consumers prefer products guaranteed pesticide-free
- whether it contains anything that could be harmful.

Concerns have been raised, for example, about mineral oil ('petrolatum' or paraffinum liquidum), which can draw natural oils out of the skin – along with the fat-soluble vitamins (A, D, E and K) in them; and diethanolamine (DEA) and monoethanolamine (MEA), which can react with any nitrites present in the product to form nitrosamines that could, at worst, encourage cancer. If you don't like the idea of putting such things as petrochemicals and high concentrations of preservatives such as formaldehyde on your skin, look for vegetable-based ranges. But beware: some products are described as 'natural' simply because a tiny amount of a plant extract, for example, has been added. An alternative is to make your own skin-care products (see Chapter 2) so you know exactly what you are putting on your skin.

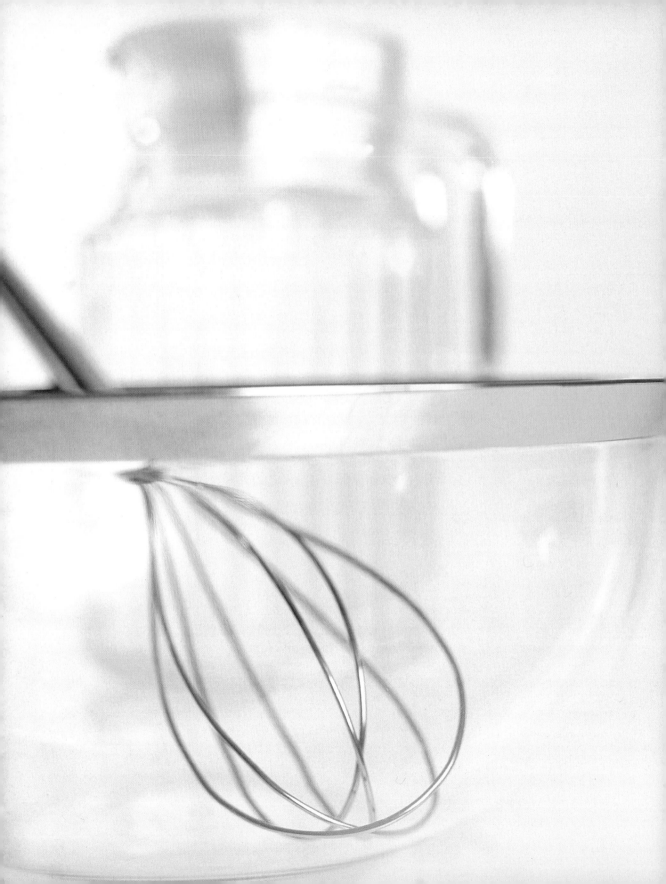

making your own products

Give almost any woman an expensive, beautifully wrapped skin-care product and she will know it's a luxury. She will also know the wrapping, box, label, pot, marketing and retail space account for much of its price. But the odds are high that she will be delighted by its mystique and the implicit promise of beauty it brings.

However, give that same woman the right ingredients, pans, utensils and guidance for her to make her own skin-care products and she may surprise herself by thoroughly enjoying the experiment. For making your own moisturiser, lip balm or eye gel will remind you of when you were a child playing. Mixing fragrant essential oils is both intriguing and enjoyable. And the resulting products are lovely to use, free from unwanted additives and much cheaper than their shop-bought equivalents.

why make your own skin-care products?

Having fun in the kitchen by stirring pans and bowls of skin-care ingredients is great fun for anyone who likes either 'cooking' or generally messing about with their hands on. Quite apart from the fact that the very process of preparing home-made skin-care products is enjoyable, there's the added advantage that you end up with a finished product formulated with the ingredients you have chosen especially for your skin. It may also be cheaper than its shop-bought equivalent.

If you have a go, you'll find that onlookers of all ages, from young children to grandmothers, are generally fascinated by the very idea of making such things at home. And they are often eager to have a go themselves. But what if your life is already packed with things to do?

Paradoxically, making some of your own skin products – perhaps a fragrant, rose-scented moisturizing cream, a cooling, aloe-based eye gel, or a gentle, brightening oatmeal skin rub – could be just the thing you need to counteract the challenges and strains of modern everyday life. For it will give you the chance to focus on yourself, on your needs and those of your skin; it will also allow you to switch off the critical, decision-making left side of your brain and let the more creative, hedonistic right side take over. The combination of the pleasure and intrinsic stress relief of the process, together with the delight of using the finished product in the hours, days or weeks to come, is almost guaranteed to bring a smile to your eyes, relax any undue tension in your scalp, shoulders and back, and bring a real lift to your face.

Another bonus is making extra to give as presents. You might want to be especially creative with their presentation by, for example, choosing an unusual container, writing the label in coloured copperplate writing, using an outer wrapper of crisp new cellophane, and tying it up with a bow of thin ribbon or husky string.

CHOOSING WHAT TO MAKE

Once you have decided what sort of a product to start with, you can choose your recipe. Some of those in this chapter suit every skin type; others are indicated for normal, dry, oily or mature skin. If you have 'combination' skin (with an oily T-zone down the centre of your face), you may find it better to use separate products for the drier and the oilier areas.

You may well have some of the ingredients already in your cupboards, fridge and, perhaps, bathroom and garden. If not, most are available at supermarkets, pharmacies or health stores; you can obtain beeswax from health stores, or from beekeepers or candlemaking suppliers (address in phone directory).

EQUIPMENT

The full kit you will need for making skin-care products at home includes:

- **sterilized glass or ceramic jars of assorted sizes with screw- on or other lids**
- **sterilized misting spray bottles**
- **labels**
- **glass or china mixing bowls**
- **measuring jug**

- **cheese grater**
- **blender**
- **sharp knife and chopping board**
- **pestle and mortar**
- **balloon whisk**
- **wooden spoon**
- **tablespoons (15 ml spoons) and teaspoons (5 ml spoons)** *(in the following recipes these are level measures unless otherwise stated)*
- **double boiler (as for making porridge) or a proper 'bain-marie' – a rounded-bottom, metal bowl that fits into the top of a pan of simmering water for heating easily**

burnable ingredients

(alternatively, stand a heatproof glass bowl in the pan, fill with water to about a third of the way up the bowl and make sure there is plenty of room around it)

SOME BASIC INGREDIENTS

Most basic ingredients are available from supermarkets, pharmacies or health stores, by special order if necessary. Some of the plant oils and extracts used in commercially produced skin-care products and home-made recipes were mentioned on page 29. Here are some reasons for choosing the other ingredients:

Almonds: soften; soothe; provide vitamin E; exfoliate

Apple cider vinegar: has a similar acidity to that of skin

Apricot kernel oil: softens; heals; moisturizes

Banana: soothes; softens

Beeswax: prevents oils separating out in creams and lotions

Borage (starflower) oil: softens; soothes; moisturizes

Cucumber: soothes; tightens

Egg: tightens (especially the white); moisturizes (especially the yolk)

Evening primrose oil: moisturizes

Frankincense oil: said to promote skin-cell regeneration

Glycerine: moisturizes by attracting water from air; improves texture of creams and lotions

Grapefruit juice: tightens;

counteracts infection

Lemon peel: tightens; lightens; soothes; counteracts infection

Milk: soothes; moisturizes; tightens; brightens by exfoliating

Mint: tightens; freshens

Neroli oil: soothes

Oatmeal: soothes; lightens; brightens by exfoliating; provides vitamin E

Olive oil: softens; soothes

Parsley: tightens; counteracts infection

Rose water: promotes regeneration; tightens; counteracts infection

Sugar: brightens by exfoliating; tightens; counteracts infection

Yoghurt: soothes; moisturizes; tightens; brightens by exfoliating

AFTERCARE OF PRODUCTS

Put each skin-care product you make into a lidded container that you have first sterilized by rinsing it inside with boiling water. Try to use a container of the correct size so the air space inside is as small as possible and lay a waxed-paper disc directly on to the surface of the product (as for home-made jam) if it is of a thick enough consistency to support one – these measures will help to keep it fresh. Home-made products have the advantage that they don't need as long a shelf-life as commercial products, because you can start using them as soon as they are made. This means that many can be preservative-free and others can be made with natural preservatives, such as honey, vinegar or vitamin E. It is therefore best to store them in the fridge or, at least, in a cool, dark place. Make only a small quantity of those products that contain no preservative so that you can use them up quickly.

CLEANSERS

Lemon-herbal steam cleansing for all skin types

- **Boiling water**
- **Peel from ½ lemon (full thickness – both yellow and white parts)**
- **1 teaspoon dried or 2 heaped teaspoons chopped fresh mint**
- **1 teaspoon dried or 2 heaped teaspoons chopped parsley**
- **Optional extra for dry skin – contents of 1 capsule evening primrose oil**

Three-quarters fill a 1.2-litre (2-pint/5-cup) bowl with boiling water and add the lemon peel, mint, parsley and, if you wish, the evening primrose oil. Sit at a table with your face over the bowl in front of you and cover your head and the bowl with a towel to prevent steam from escaping.

Enjoy this fragrant facial sauna for five minutes, then splash your face with lukewarm water.

Lavender cleanser for oily skin

- **2 tablespoons grated beeswax**
- **1 tablespoon sweet-almond oil**
- **2 drops lavender oil**
- **1 tablespoon mineral water**

Melt the beeswax in a double boiler or bain-marie (see page 33). Remove from the heat and beat in the almond oil, lavender oil and water until creamy. Use within two weeks. Smooth into your skin with clean fingers, then gently remove with cotton wool or a soft paper tissue.

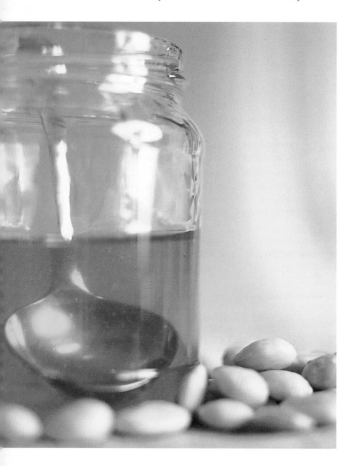

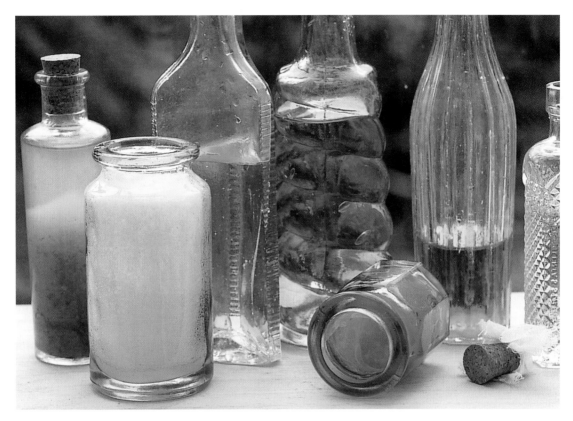

Honey-almond cleanser for all skin types

- **6 tablespoons almonds, brought to the boil in water, cooled and skinned**
- **2 teaspoons honey**
- **200ml (7fl oz/scant 1 cup) mineral water**
- **4 tablespoons rose water**

Blend the almonds, honey and mineral water. Leave overnight in the fridge, then put the mixture in the middle of a clean square of muslin, bring the free edges together and twist them round. Squeeze the almond milk into a bowl. Add the rose water. Use within two weeks. Apply with cotton wool and remove by splashing your face with warm water or gently wiping off with cotton wool, a soft paper tissue or a moistened face flannel.

Foaming soapwort wash

- **1 tablespoon soapwort root (*from a health store or herbal supplier*)**
- **2 tablespoons dried or 4 heaped tablespoons chopped fresh herb (*rosemary, chamomile, lime flowers or nettle for normal skin; lemon peel, sage, mint or lavender flowers for oily; parsley, borage or chamomile for dry*)**
- **1.5 litres (2¹/₂ pints/6¹/₄ cups) mineral water**

If using lemon peel, use the full thickness – both yellow and white parts. Put the soapwort, herb or lemon peel and water in a pan, bring to the boil, cover and simmer for five minutes. Pour the mixture into a bowl, cool and strain using a sieve, pushing as much herby 'soapwort tea' as possible through with a wooden spoon. Use within three weeks.

Herbal milk cleanser

- **2 tablespoons dried or 4 heaped tablespoons chopped fresh herb (*rosemary, chamomile, lime flowers or nettle for normal skin; lemon peel, sage, mint or lavender flowers for oily; parsley, borage or chamomile for dry*)**
- **300ml (1/2 pint/11/4 cups) whole milk**

If using lemon peel, use the full thickness – both the yellow and the white parts. If using a dried herb, preheat the milk to below boiling point, remove from heat and add the herb. If using a fresh herb or lemon peel, add it to cold milk. Cover, soak for four hours in a cool place, then strain, using a sieve and pushing as much milk as possible through with a wooden spoon. The milk will be slightly coloured. Apply with cotton wool and remove by splashing your face with warm water or gently wiping off with clean cotton wool, a soft paper tissue or a moistened flannel. Use within three days.

FLOWER AND HERB FRESHENERS TO SPLASH OR MIST ON THE SKIN

Lavender water for all skin types

- **6 drops lavender oil**
- **120ml (4 fl oz/1/2 cup) mineral water**

Place the lavender oil and mineral water in a sterilized screw-top jar, put the lid on tightly and shake well. Transfer to a sterilized bottle or spray bottle. Use within two weeks.

Cypress water

As for lavender water in the above recipe, using cypress oil instead of lavender oil.

Apple cider vinegar splash for all skin types

- **1 tablespoon apple cider vinegar**
- **120ml (4 fl oz/1/2 cup) mineral water**

Place the apple cider vinegar and water in a sterilized screw-top jar, put the lid on tightly and shake well. Transfer to a sterilized bottle or spray bottle. Use within two weeks.

Herbal tea

- **Boiling water**
- **1 teaspoon dried or 2 heaped teaspoons chopped fresh herb (*rosemary, chamomile, lime flowers or nettle for normal skin; lemon peel, sage, mint or lavender flowers for oily; parsley, borage or chamomile for dry*)**

If using lemon peel, use the full thickness – both yellow and white parts. Put the herb or lemon peel in a cup and cover with boiling water. Steep until cold, then strain through a sieve. Transfer to a sterilized bottle or spray bottle. Use within three days.

Rose water and witch hazel for oily skin

- **1 tablespoon witch hazel**
- **1 tablespoon rose water**

Place the witch hazel and rose water into a sterilized screw-top jar, put the lid on tightly and shake well. Transfer to a sterilized bottle or spray bottle. Use within two weeks.

MOISTURIZERS

Increase the hydrating power of a moisturizer by first splashing or misting some water, lavender water or herbal tea on your face, then applying the moisturizer to still-damp skin to seal in a fine layer of water.

Custom-made cream

- 1 tablespoon beeswax

- 3 tablespoons vegetable oil (such as one or more of the following: olive, rapeseed/canola, wheatgerm, sweet almond, jojoba, sunflower, evening primrose, borage/starflower)

- 1 tablespoon lavender water or herbal tea (see page 36)

- 3 drops essential oil (lavender, ylang ylang, geranium, neroli, rose, jasmine, clary sage or chamomile for normal or dry skin; lavender, neroli, sandalwood, cypress, juniper berry, cedarwood or cardamom for oily)

- contents of 1 capsule vitamin E

Melt the beeswax in a double boiler or bain-marie, then slowly beat in the vegetable oil. Remove from the heat and slowly beat in the lavender water or herbal tea. Carry on stirring until the cream is lukewarm, then stir in the essential oil and vitamin E. Use within two weeks.

Honey cream smoother

- 1 tablespoon beeswax

- 1 tablespoon any scented honey (such as clover or acacia)

- 2 tablespoons *Custom-made cream* (see above)

Melt the beeswax in a double boiler or bain-marie, then remove from the heat and stir in the honey. When lukewarm, stir in the cream. Use within two weeks.

Glycerine and neroli for dry skin

- 1 teaspoon glycerine

- 1 tablespoon mineral water

- 3 drops neroli oil

Place the glycerine, water and neroli oil into a small sterilized screw-top jar, put the lid on tightly and shake well. Use within two weeks.

Oil-free moisturizer for oily skin

- 1 teaspoon dried or 2 heaped teaspoons chopped fresh sage or mint leaves or lavender or marigold flowers

- 6 tablespoons mineral water

- 50ml (2 fl oz/¼ cup) rose water

- 2 tablespoons glycerine

- 2 tablespoons witch hazel

Put the herbs in a pan, add the water, bring to the boil and simmer for ten minutes. Cool, strain through a sieve, then add the rose water, glycerine and witch hazel. Place in a sterilized screw-top jar, put the lid on tightly and shake well. Use within three days.

EYEMAKE-UP REMOVER

Gentle jojoba eye make-up remover

- 4 tablespoons jojoba oil

- 5 drops calendula (marigold) tincture

Place the jojoba oil and calendula tincture into a small sterilized screw-top jar, put the lid on tightly and shake well. Use within three weeks. Smooth on to your eyelids with a cotton pad or cotton wool and remove with one or more fresh pads or pieces of cotton wool. Repeat if necessary.

LIP SALVES

Honey lip saver

- 2 tablespoons beeswax

- 4 tablespoons sweet-almond oil

- 2 teaspoons honey

Melt the beeswax in a double boiler or bain-marie, remove from the heat, then stir in the almond oil and honey. Use within six weeks.

Lavender lip saver

- **2 tablespoons beeswax**
- **1 tablespoon apricot kernel oil**
- **1 tablespoon wheatgerm oil**
- **3 drops lavender oil**

Melt the beeswax in a double boiler or bain-marie, remove from the heat, then stir in the apricot kernel and wheatgerm oils. When lukewarm, stir in the lavender oil. Use within six weeks.

YOUTH DEWS

Milk and honey marvel

- **25g (1 oz) honey**
- **175ml (6 fl oz/³/₄ cup) milk**

Put the honey in a double boiler or bain-marie and warm it up a little. Remove from the heat and stir in the milk. Cool. Use within three days. Apply with a cotton pad or cotton wool, leave for fifteen to thirty minutes, rinse off with warm water, pat almost dry, then apply moisturizer.

Cucumber lifter

- **15cm (6 in) length cucumber, cut into thick slices**

Put the cucumber in a blender and liquidize. Use immediately. Smooth over your skin with clean fingers, leave for fifteen to thirty minutes, rinse off with warm water, pat almost dry, then apply moisturizer.

HOLDING BACK THE YEARS

Looking young often goes hand in hand with being sexually attractive, enjoying good health, and having a high chance of employment. So not surprisingly many people continue to seek the elixir of youth as they grow older. Trying to discover the perfect face cream, lotion or other potion is a popular part of this search. Many skin-care ingredients suitable for home-made products can help prevent or disguise premature skin ageing. Here are some of the best.

Anti-oxidants

- Wheatgerm oil
- Carrot oil
- Ground almonds
- Oatmeal

Moisturizers

- Apricot kernel oil
- Borage (starflower) oil
- Jojoba oil

Soothers

- Olive oil
- Roman chamomile oil
- Yoghurt

Plant-hormone-rich oils

- Clary sage oil
- Roman chamomile oil

Skin cell regenerators

- Frankincense oil
- Neroli oil
- Rosa mosqueta oil
- Rose water

Skin tighteners

- Lemon juice and peel
- Honey
- Cucumber
- Egg white

A simple smoother

- 2 tablespoons sweet-almond oil
- 2 teaspoons honey
- 1 teaspoon apple cider vinegar
- 1 tablespoon plain yoghurt

Put all the ingredients in a bowl and mix well. Use within three days. Apply as for *Milk and honey marvel* (above).

A fragrant oil

- 1 tablespoon jojoba oil
- 1 tablespoon rapeseed (canola) oil
- 1 teaspoon extra-virgin olive oil
- contents of 1 capsule borage (starflower) oil
- 5 drops neroli oil
- 3 drops frankincense oil
- 3 drops lavender oil

Place all the oils in a sterilized screw-top jar, put the lid on tightly and shake well. Use within six weeks. Smooth a little into your skin at night after applying moisturizer.

SUNSCREENS

Several vegetable substances can help protect skin from sun damage by mopping up some of the UV rays. These include carrot seed and carrot root oil, avocado oil, shea butter and aloe vera gel. Their SPF is very low – that of shea butter is 4, for example – but it could be worth including one of them in a winter moisturizer formula.

EXFOLIATER

A slice of apple or papaya gently rubbed over the skin will help lift loose cells, as will all the following recipes:

- 1 tablespoon fine oatmeal with enough whole milk, herbal tea, honey or grape juice to make a firm paste
- 1 tablespoon ground almonds with enough natural bio yoghurt or rose water to make a firm paste
- 1 tablespoon caster sugar moistened with enough of your usual cream or milk cleanser, or moisturizer, to make a firm paste

EYE GEL/PADS/CREAM

Herby almond gel to soften lines around the eyes

- 1 teaspoon aloe vera gel
- 1 teaspoon herbal tea (see page 36)
- 1 teaspoon ground almonds

Mix all the ingredients together. Use within three days. Smooth into the skin above and below your eyes half an hour before applying make-up, then rinse off with warm water.

Cucumber cooler

- 7.5cm (3 in) length cucumber
- 2 teaspoons aloe vera gel

Put the cucumber and aloe vera gel in a blender and liquidize. Use at once to moisten two cotton eye pads. Place one over each closed eye and leave for fifteen to thirty minutes.

Soothing eye cream

- 2 teaspoons wheatgerm oil
- 2 teaspoons any moisturizer
- 1 teaspoon herbal tea (see page 36) made with eyebright (*you can use the rest of the tea you make as a refreshing splash for your whole face*)

Put all ingredients in a bowl; mix well. Use within three days.

MASKS

Many fruits and vegetables make excellent moisturizing masks. Choose from bananas, strawberries, peaches, apples, grapefruit, lemons, papayas, avocados and watercress. To make the mask, simply mash, finely chop or liquidize your chosen item and smooth it over your skin. Lie down for ten to twenty minutes, then wash off, pat dry and apply some moisturizer (see pages 36–7 for moisturizer recipes).

Citrus lifter

- **1 egg white, well beaten**
- **1 teaspoon egg yolk**
- **1 tablespoon freshly squeezed grapefruit juice**
- **1 drop from a vitamin E capsule**

Mix together the egg white, egg yolk, grapefruit juice and vitamin E. Use within twenty-four hours.

Yoghurt-banana-honey mask

- **1/2 banana**
- **1 tablespoon honey**
- **2 tablespoons plain set bio yoghurt**

Mash the banana and then add the honey and yoghurt and mix them all together so that they form a smooth paste. Use within two hours.

Herbal mask

- **1 handful dried or 2 handfuls fresh herb (*rosemary, chamomile, lime flowers or nettle for normal skin; sage, mint or lavender flowers for oily; parsley or chamomile for dry*)**

If using a dried herb, put it in a bowl, cover with boiling water and pound for one minute. Leave to stand for several hours, then strain through a sieve. If using a fresh herb, liquidize it with 1–2 tablespoons water, then strain off any surplus water. Use immediately.

COMPRESSES AND PATCHES

For a soothing compress to refresh and moisturize skin, soak a face flannel or piece of soft, clean, cotton material in lavender water or herbal tea (see page 36); or in equal quantities of rose water and mineral water mixed together. Lightly wring out compress, lie down and lay it over your face. Relax for twenty to thirty minutes, then remove it and apply some moisturizer.

If you like this treatment and plan to repeat it often, make a specially shaped compress by cutting an oval piece of soft cotton towelling large enough to overlap the edges of your face. Cut holes in your compress for your nose and eyes.

While wearing your compress, soothe your eyelids and the skin around your eyes with the moisturizing, depuffing effects of a moist teabag, or a slice of melon or cucumber. If you cool them in the refrigerator first you will find that they will feel even more refreshing.

Anti-wrinkle patches

- **175ml (6 fl oz/3/4 cup) room temperature mineral water**
- **3 drops geranium, rose, neroli or clary sage oil**
- **cotton pads**

Put the water in a bowl and add the oil. Lay each pad, one at a time, on the surface of the water to pick up some of the floating layer of oil. Lie down and apply this side of the pad as a patch over an area of lined skin. Relax for forty-five minutes, then remove and apply some moisturizer.

Anti-ageing aromatherapy compress

- **175 ml (6 fl oz/3/4 cup) lukewarm mineral water**
- **1 teaspoon avocado (or olive) oil**
- **3 drops rose oil**
- **2 drops geranium oil**
- **Face-flannel (wash-cloth) or face-sized piece of cotton cloth**

Put the water in a large shallow bowl and add the oils. Lay the face-flannel, or cotton cloth, over the surface of the water so it picks up some of the floating layer of oils, then squeeze gently. Lie down and place the flannel, or cloth, over your face, oily side down. Relax for about forty-five minutes, then remove and apply some moisturizer.

'Lipstick-line' eraser patches

- **1 teaspoon glycerine**
- **1 teaspoon rose water**
- **3 drops apricot kernel oil**
- **cotton pad, cut in half**

Put the glycerine, rose water and apricot kernel oil into a small bowl and stir well. Spread a teaspoon of the mixture over one side of one of the cotton-pad halves. Lie down and lay the pad above your upper lip, moist side down. Relax for around forty-five minutes, then remove and apply some moisturizer.

'Frownie' patches

- **50 ml (2 fl oz/1/4 cup) rose water**
- **2 drops frankincense oil**
- **50 g (2 oz) ground almonds**
- **contents of 1 vitamin E capsule**
- **cotton pads**

Put the water in a bowl and add the oil. Stir in the ground almonds and vitamin E to make a paste. Smooth half a teaspoon of this paste over the centre of a cotton pad. Lay the pad, paste-side down, over your frown lines. Relax for about forty-five minutes, then remove and apply moisturizer (see pages 36–7 for moisturizer recipes). Keep any leftover paste in a covered container in the fridge for up to forty-eight hours.

Gentle healing patches for scars

- **1 tablespoon aloe vera gel – preferably squeezed from a growing aloe vera plant**
- **1 teaspoon rose-hip oil**
- **1 teaspoon carrot oil**
- **contents of 1 capsule of vitamin E oil**
- **cotton pads**

Put the aloe vera gel, rose-hip oil, carrot oil and vitamin E oil into a small bowl, and mix well. Now smooth a teaspoon of this mixture over one side of a cotton pad. Lie down and lay the pad over the scar, moist side down. Relax for about forty-five minutes, then remove and apply some moisturizer (see pages 36–7 for moisturizer recipes). Keep any leftover mixture in a covered container in the fridge for up to forty-eight hours.

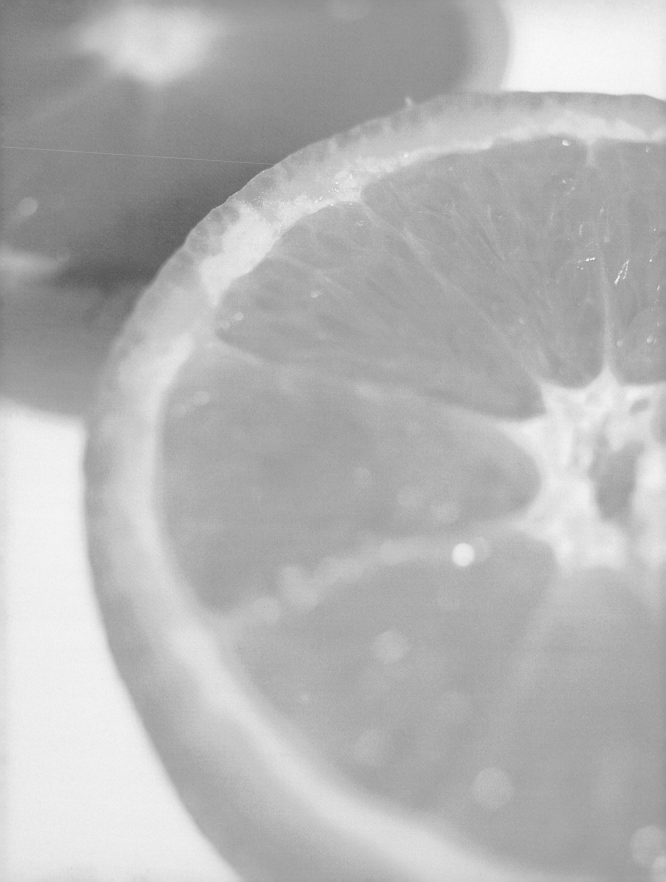

nourishing your face

The huge number of magazine features on skin creams and other products gives the impression that what you put *on* your skin is far more important than what you send to it from within. Yet this simply isn't so. While both are important, eating skin-friendly nutrients – and drinking water – are much more valuable for keeping skin looking good than any number of creams.

For a start, the skin's rich network of tiny blood vessels supplies skin cells with nutrient-rich blood day and night. Even if you were to apply nutrient-rich cream twice a day, the amounts of nutrients entering the skin would soon decline. And in any case not all topically applied nutrients get into the skin.

So what should we be eating and drinking if we are to be kind to our skin? Skin needs the same nutrients as the rest of your body. But certain minerals, fatty acids, and plant pigments and hormones are particularly important.

healthy eating guidelines

Have at least three meals a day, including breakfast, and choose a wide variety of whole foods in the amounts indicated below.

Eat six to eleven daily helpings of unrefined starchy carbohydrate foods, such as potatoes, rice, bread, pasta and cereal. A helping is half a cup of cooked potatoes, pasta, rice or grains; one slice of bread; or 25g (1 oz) cereal. Opt usually for wholemeal or wholegrain rice, bread and cereals, and potatoes in their jackets. Slowly digested carbohydrates – such as those in oats, beans and lentils – help maintain a good energy supply to you and your skin. These and other complex carbohydrates should provide around 50 percent of your daily calories.

Eat at least five helpings of vegetables, salads and fruit a day, including some raw. A helping is one apple or similar-sized fruit, or one small bowl of a vegetable.

Include beans, peas or lentils several times a week. Their plant oestrogens – like your own oestrogens – can latch on to oestrogen receptors on skin cells, which helps keep these cells plump and unlined. This happens in women and men, though women, of course, have higher oestrogen levels. Their effects are not as strong as those of your own oestrogens. But by latching on to empty receptors they help correct any oestrogen-progesterone imbalance resulting from a low or rapidly falling level of your own oestrogens (such as after the menopause, when they act as a mild hormone replacement therapy). And by latching on to receptors ahead of your own oestrogens, they can also counteract any oestrogen-progesterone imbalance resulting from a high level of your own

oestrogens, so discouraging irregular heavy periods, fibroids and, perhaps, some types of facial reddening and puffy eyes.

Proteins are essential for healthy skin and come from meat, poultry, fish, eggs, dairy products, peas, lentils, beans and soya bean-derived foods such as tofu and soya milk. You need two to three daily helpings – a helping being 55–85g (2–3 oz) of lean meat, poultry or seafood; one egg; or half a cup of beans. Proteins should contribute around 15 percent of daily calories.

Healthy, smooth, supple skin relies on your eating enough essential fats (linoleic acid and alpha-linolenic acid). Your body can make all the other fats it needs from nutrients other than fats if necessary, but it *must* obtain enough essential fats from your diet. An average-weight woman taking an average amount of exercise needs only 70g (2¹/₂ oz) of fats a day; an average-weight man 100g (3¹/₄ oz). And these fats should have a healthy balance. To achieve this, aim for the following.

- **30–35 percent of daily calories as fats.** The average intake in many developed countries is over 40 percent. Look at food labels: if 100g of a food contain over 20g of fats, it is a high-fat food; if under 5g, it is a low-fat one. There are 10g of fat in 100g of a '90 percent fat-free' food, so this is not a low-fat food.

- **Less than 10 per cent of daily calories as saturated fat.** The average intake is at least 17 percent. Another guide is to have only 20g a day. Lower your intake by replacing some of it with monounsaturated fat.

- **Few or no trans fats.** These have potentially harmful effects like those of saturated fats, and are present in over-heated polyunsaturated fats (PUFAs) and hard margarines.
- **A good balance of the two essential fats.** We need three times as much linoleic acid (the essential 'omega-6' PUFA) as alpha-linolenic acid (the essential 'omega-3' PUFA). But the average person consumes six times as much.

- **Two to three helpings of oily fish a week.** These are rich in two omega-3 PUFAs, docosahexaenoic acid (DHA) and eicosapentanoic acid (EPA). Although DHA and EPA are not essential for most of us (because we make them from alpha-linolenic acid), several factors – such as stress, smoking, ageing, alcohol, a lack of vitamin B6, magnesium or zinc; and too much processed and fried food – can stop you making enough.

skin-friendly nutrients

Every cell in the body needs some of each nutrient, but certain of these are particularly important for the skin.

FIBRE

This promotes a healthy hormone balance and helps to prevent constipation that can encourage dullness and sallowness of the skin.

Sources: fruit; vegetables; wholegrains; brown rice.

FATS

A good balance of dietary fats helps in a number of different ways: first it boosts immunity; second it helps prevent dry skin, rashes and skin cancer; third it promotes skin elasticity and strength by helping build collagen and elastin; and finally it fosters the production of specialized fats such as phospholipids (that help keep cell membranes healthy) in the muscles and the arteries.

Saturated fats

Sources: beef, pork and lamb; dairy products; hard margarines; white cooking fat; coconut oil; palm oil; processed fatty foods such as shop-bought biscuits and shop-bought pastry.

Trans fats

Sources: most margarines; processed fatty foods such as shop-bought biscuits and shop-bought pastry; 'partially hydrogenated oil', 'vegetable fat' or 'shortening'.

Monounsaturated fats

Sources: olives, avocados, nuts, sesame seeds and oil, rapeseed (canola) oil.

Polyunsaturated fats (PUFAs)

Sources: vegetables, seeds, nuts and their oils; wholegrains; meat (especially poultry); oily fish.

Essential PUFAs

Linoleic acid

Sources: avocados; beans; corn and its oil; seeds and seed oils; safflower oil, soya oil; wholegrains, soft margarine.

Alpha-linolenic acid

Sources: green leafy vegetables; broccoli; beans, walnuts and peanuts and their oil; pumpkin seeds and their oil; linseeds (flaxseeds); wholegrains; rapeseed (canola) oil; soya oil; sweet potatoes; chicken; meat from grass-fed animals.

CALCIUM

Together with magnesium, this nourishes nerves, muscles and blood vessels, promoting healthy skin and strong muscles.

Sources: tinned sardines or salmon (eaten with bones); shellfish; dairy products; eggs; beans; peas; lentils; nuts; seeds; wholegrains; green leafy vegetables.

MAGNESIUM

This has similar effects to those of calcium.

Sources: meat; fish; eggs; leafy green vegetables; mushrooms; beans; peas; nuts; seeds; wholegrains.

SELENIUM

This helps prevent free radicals (see page 24) ageing skin prematurely.

Sources: meat; fish; dairy products; egg yolk; leafy green vegetables; mushrooms; garlic; beans; peas; wholegrains.

SILICON

This aids collagen formation. A falling silicon level with age encourages sagging and wrinkles.

Sources: wholegrains; beans.

SULPHUR

This promotes the production of keratin and collagen. Processing reduces a food's sulphur content so where possible buy natural, unprocessed foods; our sulphur level also falls with age.

Sources: meat; fish; dairy products; garlic; onions; beans; peas; wholegrains.

ZINC

This reduces free-radical formation (see page 24) and helps prevent damage to the circulation and skin cells.

Sources: red meat; shellfish; liver; dairy products; root vegetables; small amounts in beans, peas, nuts, seeds, wholegrains, vegetables and fruit.

VITAMIN A AND BETA-CAROTENE

This promotes supple, firm, unlined skin by retaining moisture and promoting collagen and elastin production.

Sources: fish; dairy products; eggs; many fruits and vegetables, especially orange and red ones.

VITAMIN B AND FOLIC ACID

These are vital for healthy nerves, blood vessels and muscles. Vitamins B2 and B6 help skin retain moisture; B6 helps prevent puffiness; B12 encourages skin-cell renewal.

Sources: meat; fish; dairy products; eggs; beans and peas; nuts and seeds; wholegrain foods; fruit and vegetables, particularly leafy green ones and mushrooms.

VITAMIN C

This has renewing, protecting and healing effects on skin. It helps prevent clogging of the arteries with a fatty substance called atheroma (which diminishes the skin's oxygen and nutrient supply); helps counteract free-radical damage by sun, pollution and smoking; improves skin resilience and strength; helps with scar repair by stimulating collagen formation; and reduces inflammation.

Sources: fruit, especially citrus and kiwis; vegetables.

VITAMIN D

This helps us to absorb and to use both calcium and magnesium.

Sources: our major source is from sunlight on the skin; it is also available from butter, cheese and other full-fat dairy produce; eggs; oily fish.

VITAMIN E

Vitamin E's antioxidant action prolongs cell life and improves skin quality by destroying free radicals (see page 24). It also helps protect against sun damage (and may even partially reverse it) and encourages the skin to retain moisture. Finally, it reduces scar formation.

Sources: meat; fish; dairy products; eggs; leafy green vegetables; beans; peas; nuts; seeds; wholegrain foods.

FLAVONOIDS

These plant pigments may help foster a healthy blood supply to skin by strengthening tiny blood vessels. They work in conjunction with vitamin C.

Sources: all coloured fruits and vegetables.

OTHER PLANT PIGMENTS

Many other pigments besides flavonoids provide colour in edible roots, stems, leaves, seeds and berries. Some of these, such as proanthocyanidins and reseveratrol act as powerful anti-oxidants against free radicals.

Sources: any brightly coloured plant material; blue, purple, red and black berries; cherries; black grape skins.

PLANT HORMONES

Plant hormones help to prevent premature lines and wrinkles.

Sources: bean sprouts; fennel; celery; parsley; beans; peas; lentils; chick-peas; wholegrain foods; seeds; potatoes; carrots; beetroot; cabbage; garlic; sage; beer; cherries; plums; rhubarb; olives; and many other vegetables and fruits.

boosting the nutrient value of your food

Several everyday tips can help you gain as much benefit as possible from the skin-friendly (and other) nutrients in your food:

- Don't go food shopping when you are hungry, as hunger makes many of us choose too many foods that are high in calories from sugar and saturated fat.
- Wash fruit and vegetables to remove pesticide traces.
- Peel vegetables and fruit immediately before cooking or eating to minimize vitamin C loss.
- Eat more fresh fruit and vegetables; tinned ones don't contain as much folic acid, and vegetables blanched before being frozen may contain only a low level of vitamin C.
- Cook fruit and vegetables as little as possible to preserve vitamins B12 and C. Use the water in which you have cooked them to make a sauce, gravy or soup.
- Read labels on foods to make wise choices.
- Deep-fry only occasionally and don't re-use cooking fat more than a few times.

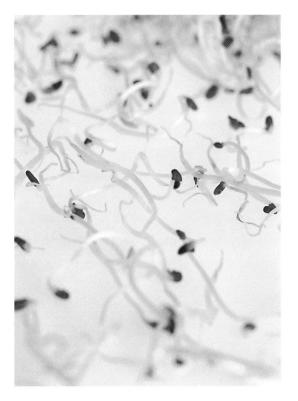

SPROUTING

An excellent way of boosting your intake of skin-friendly nutrients – yet one that is little used other than in Asian communities – is to sprout beans and seeds at home. This boosts their content of plant hormones, beta-carotene, vitamins B, C and E, enzymes and minerals such as calcium, iron, silicon and zinc.

Sprouting means encouraging them to start growing roots and shoots. Do this by soaking a tablespoonful or so of the seeds in water overnight, draining them, then rinsing and draining twice a day for however long it takes them to form sprouts of the size you want. Alfalfa seeds are very easy to sprout and taste delicious. Mung beans are good too, and if you keep them relatively dark and weigh them down with something heavy as they grow, you will end up with the fat, white sprouts that are so popular with Chinese cooks.

DRINKS

Our skin needs adequate amounts of water for its cells to remain plump and to enable it to appear as smooth and unlined as possible, because water forms the bulk of each living skin cell. The quantity we need depends on how big and active we are, as well as on our health and on the flow, temperature and humidity of the surrounding air. However, we can tolerate wide variations in the volume we drink because our kidneys and sweat glands regulate the amount of fluid in our body so efficiently. If we drink a lot, we produce larger quantities of urine (unless we are dehydrated and need to restore our fluid level). If we drink only a little, we produce smaller amounts of more concentrated urine.

Our body can extract the water it needs from any water-based fluid, and even from many solid foods. However, some naturopaths and other alternative therapists recommend drinking relatively large quantities of water. A figure of eight to ten 300-ml (1/2 pint/1 1/4 cups) glasses a day is often mentioned. They claim this promotes good health by ensuring that the kidneys have plenty of water with which to flush waste products and toxins from the body. In contrast, most doctors believe there is no scientific backing for this advice. They say that – for most of the time, at least – we need to drink simply according to our thirst. If you don't trust your thirst as a guide, aim to drink enough to keep your urine pale yellow.

Several types of drink, including alcohol, coffee, tea and caffeinated colas, actively encourage dehydration by promoting fluid loss from the kidneys. So from your skin's point of view it is unwise to drink too much of these. Help protect yourself and your skin from dehydration by alternating each alcoholic drink, cup of tea or coffee, or glass of cola with a glass of water.

FOOD SUPPLEMENTS

It is nearly always better to get nutrients from a healthy diet than to take the same substances as food supplements. However, while good evidence for the benefits of these supplements is often lacking, it does sometimes seem wise to take certain of them.

The most effective formulations of vitamin C contain flavonoids that boost its action. The best vitamin E is the natural type, and you can boost its action by taking it with vitamin C.

- If you aren't eating enough food, take a multi-mineral and vitamin supplement.
- If you have diarrhoea, take a multi-mineral and vitamin supplement, and either live yoghurt each day or a supplement of probiotics ('friendly' bacteria that help restore a healthy population of micro-organisms in the bowel).
- If you spend much time outdoors, some evidence suggests that antioxidants – beta-carotene and vitamins C and E – may help protect your skin from sun damage.
- If you are physically or emotionally stressed, take vitamin C to lower your stress-hormone levels and safeguard your immunity.
- If you drink a lot of tea or coffee, take vitamin C to make up for the resulting depletion of this skin-friendly vitamin.
- If you continue to smoke, take extra vitamin C and folic acid.
- If you have a rash (such as rosacea), or many skin tags or moles, and already eat two helpings of oily fish a week, try a daily supplement of fish oil. This provides certain omega-3 fats (DHA and EPA, see page 45) that help counter inflammation and abnormal cell growth.

- If your skin is ageing prematurely, try a daily supplement of starflower (borage) oil or evening primrose oil for three months, and continue if your skin improves. These oils contain gamma-linolenic acid (GLA), an omega-6 fat whose level falls with age, especially in women.
- If ageing is shrinking and weakening your cheek and other face muscles, consider creatine and/or glutamine to help restore their power and bulk. We get these amino acids from meat and fish – and make them in our liver – but their levels fall as we age.

BODY WEIGHT AND SKIN

The amount of fat in the skin has a big impact on our looks. Most people look their best when their body mass index (BMI; see below) is 20–25. Too much fat can cause a double chin, jowls or other surplus folds. Too little may mean the skin drapes over muscles and bones in a way that makes us look drawn and craggy.

YOUR BMI

Work out your BMI by multiplying your height (in metres) by itself to give a 'height-squared' number and dividing your weight (in kilograms) by the result. For example:

65kg ÷ (1.7m x 1.7m) = 22.5

BE A 'PEAR', NOT AN 'APPLE'

Your BMI, however, isn't the only guide as to whether your weight is healthy. This is because overweight 'pears' – or pear-shaped people – whose fat is stored mainly around their hips and thighs, have a lower risk of artery disease than overweight 'apples' – or apple-shaped people – whose fat is stored mainly around their waist.

The narrowing of the arteries that accompanies arterial disease is bad news for the well-being of the skin, muscles and nerves of the face. So you need to be aware of both your height-waist ratio and your BMI when estimating whether your weight is okay. And this has one very important practical application to those trying to keep off lost weight (see also below): if, when you get dressed in the morning, the waist band of your trousers or skirt begins to feel unusually tight, that's a sign that your weight is beginning to be a health hazard again.

This is what your BMI indicates about your weight:

20–25: normal

25–30: overweight

30–35: obese

Over 35: very obese

LOSING WEIGHT

The best advice for shedding unwanted weight is to exercise more, eat a healthy diet, eat moderately and regularly, and manage stress effectively, without comfort eating. In the first week you could lose up to 3kg (7 lb), but most will be fluid. After that aim to lose 450-900g (1–2 lb) a week. Any more and your skin won't adapt fast enough to your changing facial contours. The result will be loose skin that develops lines, wrinkles and folds. The best cosmetic result comes from slow, steady weight loss.

Choose your daily food intake carefully. While a little 'junk-food' won't hurt, too much food high in calories and saturated fat, but low in skin-friendly nutrients, means you will go short of skin-friendly nutrients.

Remember that you must have essential fats (see page 45). If you eat a very low-fat diet, your body will try to restore the lack by making myristic acid, a saturated fatty acid that is the most hazardous to health of all saturated fats.

KEEPING OFF LOST WEIGHT

Many people find it relatively straightforward, if not easy, to lose excess weight. They say being well motivated, disciplined, and informed about the value of healthy eating, daily exercise, and effective stress-management are all important to their success. However, statistics repeatedly show that over nine in ten of those who lose weight on a slimming diet regain their lost weight in a year. So the problem isn't losing weight, but keeping it off.

Regaining previously lost kilos, or tens of kilos (pounds or stones) is an enormous disappointment. It's also a huge waste of endeavour. And, just as important, it's bad for health, because the process of putting on weight is in some ways more risky to physical and emotional well-being than is being very overweight.

This is because while a person is putting on weight, they are almost certain to be eating an unhealthy diet – one that is too high in calories, fats, saturated fat, and refined carbohydrates (foods made with white flour, such as most bread, biscuits, cakes and pastry), and too low in omega-3s, see page 45). The excess calories, fats and sugar in the blood bombard the blood vessels and pancreas, and adversely affect the levels of certain hormones, such as oestrogen. The result is a narrowing of the blood vessels by fatty atheroma; a lack of insulin (causing a raised risk of diabetes); and a liklihood of hormone imbalance problems (such as heavy periods or the polycystic ovary syndrome). Added to this is the feeling of many successful slimmers, once their weight starts rising again, that they are out of

control. Feeling out of control of anything is stressful, and in itself is bad news for the face (see Chapter 5), but it can also be a source of fear, frustration and anger. And if these emotions aren't recognized and managed effectively, they can lead to depression, and to the comfort eating that sabotages many a person's weight control.

So what can you do to help yourself become part of the five percent of successful slimmers who keep off lost weight?

Permanently changing the way you behave is a good start. You need to avoid going on a slimming diet, losing weight, then thinking, 'Yippee, I've lost weight, so now I can eat what I want again'. A good slimming diet is simply a healthy eating programme in which you lose weight by balancing your food intake and exercise level so your body is constantly very slightly short of food. You can do this by exercising more, eating less or a bit of both. Aim to lose only half to one kilo (one to two pounds) a week.

Most important, when you get to your goal weight, is not to revert to what were, previously, your 'normal' eating and exercise styles. Continue with a daily half-hour of exercise and allow yourself only a little more each day in terms of food intake. If you feel hungry before a meal, welcome the feeling, because it's a sign that your body is working properly. Though if you feel hungry just two hours after a meal, check that your meals contain enough 'slow-release' carbohydrates (such as oats and other wholegrains, beans and peas) to keep your blood-sugar level steadier for longer.

Most important, encourage and affirm your efforts and daily successes in keeping to a daily programme of healthy eating, exercise and stress-management. You are worth the effort and you deserve the best.

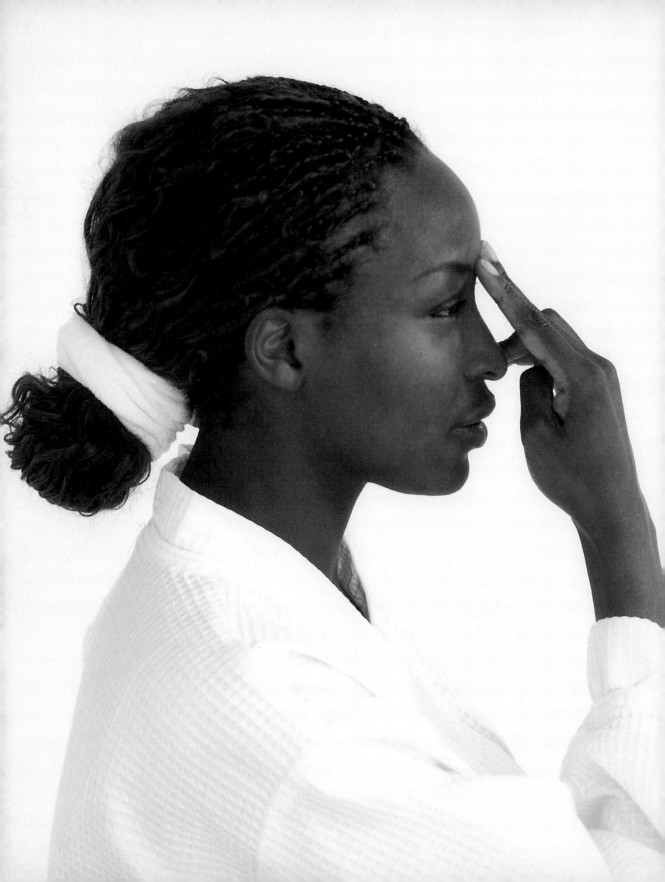

exercising
and breathing

Regular exercise is vitally important to all of us – young or old, able-bodied or disabled, sports enthusiast or would-be couch potato – and the good news is that it has amazing benefits for your face as well as for your general health. So what sort of exercise should you do to give your face a lift?

The surprising answer is that every sort you can think of has beneficial effects. Clearly specific facial exercises (see pages 58–61) will help, but so too does whole-body exercise.

As for breathing, it's vitally important that we get the right amount of good clean fresh air. This enables sufficient oxygen to reach the living cells in our skin, removes surplus carbon dioxide and generally helps to keep our skin glowing, smooth and supple.

whole-body exercise

Doing whole-body exercise will help your face stay younger and lovelier, but only if you do it wisely. Learning about the types of exercise will mean you use your exercise time in the way that is best for you. Aim to do a combination of aerobic (stamina), 'weight-training' (strength or resistance) and stretching (flexibility or suppleness) exercises.

AEROBIC EXERCISE

Aerobic exercise involves moving your body briskly enough to boost circulation, but not enough to get muscle pain. (Such pain would suggest your muscles were not getting enough oxygen, which would mean the exercise was 'anaerobic'.)

We all do this sort of exercise naturally with everyday activities such as climbing stairs, doing errands, cleaning the car and working around the house or garden. Aerobic exercise helps keep the heart, arteries and veins healthy and, if intense enough, can raise the metabolic rate (the rate at which cells burn energy) for several hours after stopping the exercise. This can use up 200–300 extra calories. Exercise also perks up your mood; maximizes brain power; helps you sleep well; boosts digestion; enhances looks; sculpts the body by reducing local fat deposits; makes several cancers less likely; and boosts immunity. All these also benefit the skin.

'Cardio' (cardiovascular) work is especially good for the circulation – and therefore the skin too. Moderate-intensity cardio work is aerobic exercise that is brisk enough to raise your heart rate to 50–75 percent of its safe maximum. Work out your safe cardio range by subtracting your age from 220, then multiplying the answer by 0.75 for the upper limit, and 0.5 for the lower limit. Start cardio work at the lower end of this range. Then gradually, over several weeks, increase your exercise level, raising its frequency before its intensity. Aim to feel a little out of breath (but never so breathless you cannot talk) and to keep your heart rate below the upper limit.

Caution: If you have any concerns about this, or if you are unfit or on any medication for your heart or blood pressure, talk to your doctor before starting a cardio programme.

Examples of moderate-intensity cardio exercise are brisk walking, gentle jogging, cycling, tennis and swimming; examples of high-intensity are fast swimming, cycling uphill, sprinting, squash and the fast section of a 'step' or other aerobics class.

Aim to do a total of at least thirty minutes of aerobic exercise (each split into two or three shorter sessions if you like) on each of five days a week; three of these half-hours should be cardio work.

'WEIGHT TRAINING'

This form of exercise involves contracting muscles against some sort of resistance. This could be your body's own weight (as with press-ups); weights held in the hand or strapped to an ankle; something you carry on your back; the resistance of a full spade when digging; or the pedals when cycling. Isometric exercise means you keep your muscles still; isotonic exercise means you shorten and elongate them against the same resistance. Both isometric and isotonic exercise increase muscle bulk, which allows you to define your shape and boost muscle power and, because more muscle burns more calories, helps you lose excess fat. Some people find that having a stronger body helps them feel more active, assertive and in control of their life – all positive attributes that can reflect in their face.

Aim to do some muscle-strengthening exercise at least twice a week, and preferably every other day. This allows your muscles to recover between workouts.

STRETCHING

Stretching fully extends the fibres in your big muscles to their maximum length. This irons out tension; keeps muscles, tendons and joints flexible and capable of their whole range of movement; improves balance and posture; and releases muscle tension. The result is that your body feels well conditioned, and you feel brighter and better, which has positive effects on your skin. Examples of stretching exercise include some yoga postures (asanas), reaching for the ball in tennis or badminton, and doing the crawl when swimming.

Aim to do some stretching exercise most, if not all, days of the week.

HOW WHOLE-BODY EXERCISE BENEFITS YOUR FACE

The boost to the circulation and to your natural 'feel-good' hormone-like chemicals called endorphins, combined with a reduction in muscle tension and joint stiffness, can work wonders on the face. Depending on what sort of exercise you do, and how much you do of it, you will be delighted by a whole host of benefits to the way you look. These are some of the things you may notice:

- Your face will look brighter and better, because the increased blood-flow throughout the whole body brings a glow to the cheeks, and the raised levels of endorphins lift your mood.

- You'll have clearer, healthier skin, due to the increased supply of nutrients and oxygen and faster removal of carbon dioxide and other acidic waste products.

- Your frownlines will become less pronounced, because exercise helps to counteract the feeling of being over-stressed and so relaxes stress-induced muscle tension.

- The contours of your face will become smoother, because regular aerobic exercise, combined with a healthy diet, counteracts fluid retention and reduces stores of excess fat.

- The muscles that give the contours to your face will also retain their natural fullness and withstand the tendency to shrink as you age, because facial muscle 'weight training' helps them maintain their bulk.

- Your face will be less easily fatigued, because facial muscle 'weight-training' helps boost their strength and 'lastability'.

- Your skin will be much less likely to age prematurely, because feeling, because exercise promotes a good supply of nutrients and oxygen and the faster removal of carbon dioxide and other waste products. However, smoking and excessive sun exposure can counteract this particular benefit if you're not careful.

choosing your whole-body exercise

Three steps can help you plan your weekly exercise schedule and choose what is best for you.

The first is to include all three basic forms of exercise: aerobic, stretching and 'weight training'. This is important for your body (see pages 54–5) and your face (see page 55), though most facial-exercise gurus describe only aerobic and stretching exercise, and miss out strength work.

The second – and vital – step is to promise you will let yourself choose another sort of exercise if necessary. This is not as silly as it sounds, because missing this step is responsible for many erstwhile exercisers failing to stick with their programme. If you don't like your first choice – or get

bored with it – don't let that put you off trying other types. The road to success is paved with failure. Anyway, deciding you don't like something isn't a failure – it simply means you are aware of your likes and dislikes and prepared to be assertive, realistic and determined. So try something else instead. There are hundreds of different ways of exercising your body, at least one of which is bound to be attractive enough to make you want to carry on with it (at least for some time, until you try the next thing!). All you need do is discover what this is by experimentation. This search can in itself be fun…if you let it.

The third step in choosing what exercise to do is to decide the best time of day for doing it, then to programme it into your diary so other things are less likely to crowd it out. You could even write it in red ink, or capitals, or both, so it assumes greater importance in your mind. After all, taking regular exercise – for both body and face – should be a priority in your life, along with your basic routines such as eating, drinking and sleeping.

Remember that even if you choose your exercise carefully and programme it into your diary, you won't keep it up if it doesn't fit easily and smoothly into your schedule. This means it has to be at a location readily accessible to your home or work. If you have a busy life, there's no point in choosing a gym or a swimming pool, for example, that's

HOW ABOUT TRYING:

Walking – the most popular exercise.

Swimming – at your local leisure centre.

Dancing – such as salsa, tap, Irish, line, flamenco, belly, ballet or jazz.

Yoga – the main types in the west are ashtanga (more active) and hatha (more meditative). Although originally a Hindu system of mental, physical and spiritual training, anyone can use it.

Cycling – on or off road.

T'ai chi – a gentle exercise that aids relaxation and promotes mental and physical strength and balance.

forty-five minutes away, because getting there and back would be so time-consuming that you would very soon find excuses not to go. Also, the stress of commuting could counteract some of the benefits of exercise. So clearly the answer is to look locally.

Another vital consideration is whether you like to exercise alone or in company. If you're a 'people person', then going for solitary walks each day might not be to your liking. And if you're basically a loner, you might not enjoy the intrinsic camaraderie that goes, for example, with being in a tennis club.

SOME EXERCISE TIPS

- See your doctor before starting an exercise programme if you are unfit, overweight or have high blood pressure, diabetes or heart or lung disease.
- Check the qualifications of your instructor.
- Check you eat enough carbohydrates by aiming for six to eleven daily servings of root vegetables, wholegrain foods, beans and bananas (see also page 44). This provides readily available stores of fuel in your liver and muscles, and makes you less likely to tire easily.
- Start each session with a few minutes of low-intensity exercise to warm your major muscle groups. This makes muscles more flexible and less prone to damage from strength or stretching work. It also helps prevent post-exercise stiffness or cramp.
- After warming up, stretch out the major muscle groups one by one; tense muscles are more likely to be damaged during exercise.
- Keep well hydrated, particularly during aerobic or strength exercise, because dehydration makes muscles

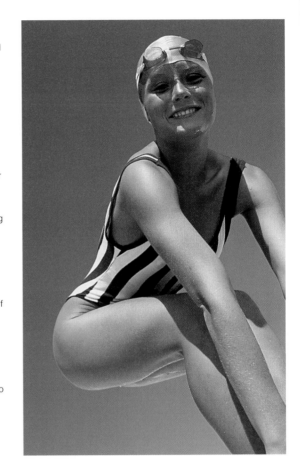

more damage-prone. Have half a glass of water at the outset, then a similar volume every 20 minutes or so. Before a long session, make your own sports drink from half fruit juice, half water, and add a small pinch of salt for each 300ml ($1/2$ pint/$1^1/4$ cups).

- If you feel hungry, eat a banana.
- As you draw your exercise to an end, gradually reduce its intensity, then repeat the initial stretching (see above).
- Aim to have no more than a light snack within two hours of starting exercise, and afterwards delay eating for at least one hour, preferably two.

exercising your face

The complexity of the face muscles is such that it's easy to understand how each person's face can be so different. And along with our bones – which we cannot alter – our facial muscles are a major determinant of how we look.

This is because their shape, bulk and tone contribute to the contours of our face. Also, while many of the facial muscles are attached to bone, some are attached to the skin itself, which means that altering their well-being has even more of a potential influence on the appearance of the skin and therefore on the way we look. Luckily there is much we can do to help them make us look as good as possible.

A healthy diet gives muscles the nutrients they need to work well and not be unnecessarily tense; those most likely to be lacking in the average person's diet are calcium, magnesium and vitamin D. Effective stress management helps prevent unnecessary tension and maintain a good circulation. Regular whole-body exercise keeps muscles fit and safeguards their blood supply, and exercises for the face itself have particular benefits.

The face contains 120 muscles and needs the three basic types of exercise – aerobic, stretching and 'weight training' – to look its relaxed, fit, glowing, youthful best. You can combine these in one daily workout or, if you want to tone one particular part of your face, concentrate on that instead. It's wise to include your neck because tension here can be reflected in the face, and any excess fat in a double chin can draw attention away from the rest of the face.

FACE AEROBICS

This involves repeatedly contracting and relaxing certain muscles, which boosts their circulation and that of the overlying skin. It also helps to reduce local fluid retention, disperse a local surplus of fat and prevent unnecessary muscle tension. A daily session will improve the way your face feels and looks and make you feel brighter and better by raising your blood levels of endorphins.

We all do face aerobics without thinking as we speak, chew, kiss and express our feelings. But sometimes certain muscles get left out – for example, if our face is tense because we are stressed, or if the face is relatively expressionless for hours in each waking day – perhaps because we are lonely, bored or depressed.

FACE STRETCHES

These release superfluous tension, helping guard against lines and folds in the overlying skin, and tension-related jaw-joint pain (temporo-mandibular joint – or TMJ – dysfunction). It also reminds you what your face feels like when it isn't tight. Many of us tense certain of our face muscles when we are feeling stressed. This not only increases our anxiety level, but the tension may stay with us when the stress is over. So relaxing your facial muscles with some stretches can be very helpful both when you are stressed and when you are not.

'WEIGHT TRAINING'

This boosts the power and bulk of certain face muscles, so strengthening them and building their bulk. This, in turn, helps to prevent facial fatigue, iron out unwanted lines and wrinkles and alter the contours of the face.

PARTNERS IN FUN

Most people who do facial exercises do so on their own, as part of their daily routine – just as they'd clean their teeth or brush their hair on their own. But if you're looking to find ways of welcoming them into your daily routine, you might sometimes like to do them with a friend, or someone in your family, because that will double their amusement value.

For the fact is that when you look at yourself in a mirror as you do these exercises, what you see as you pull faces and work the different groups of facial muscles is intrinsically a funny sight. So it's highly likely that you'll have a good laugh at yourself at some stage. And if you can share the

experience with a friend who is doing the same thing, you may find that you both enjoy yourselves even more. Having a laugh is an excellent way of boosting your spirits and making you feel better about life. This is partly because it boosts the levels of natural 'feel-good' endorphins. It also aids healing, increases immunity and educes the levels of stress hormones. So all in all, whether it's triggered by doing facial exercises or from finding amusement in some other way, laughter is an excellent therapy for both mind and body. Also, working out with a friend could help you both recognize how well you are doing with your exercises and it's likely that you will both feel the benefits of this mutual affirmation. For, as with all types of self-improvement programme, it's always wise to acknowledge your progress and to affirm any improvements that you have made.

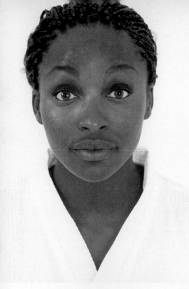

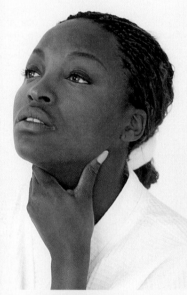

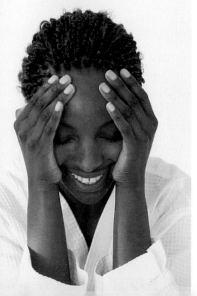

a workout for your face

The first few times you give your face a workout, sit yourself comfortably down in front of the mirror, send everyone away – unless you're happy for them to have a good laugh – and do the following sets of aerobic, 'weight training', and stretching exercises. Choose the number of repetitions according to your facial fitness level. And enjoy!

FACE AEROBICS

Smile aerobics *(top left)*

Open your mouth slightly, then smile repeatedly once a second. There's no need to smile with your eyes.

Repeat fifteen to thirty times.

'Eyes-wide-open' aerobics *(centre left)*

Raise your upper lids and eyebrows to open your eyes as wide as possible at a rate of once a second.

Repeat ten to twenty times.

Neck aerobics *(bottom left)*

Cock your head up by 45 degrees and open your mouth slightly. Rest your thumb and forefinger one either side of your neck, in the angle between the neck and lower jaw, and beneath the middle of each side of the lower jaw. Tense the underlying muscles while slightly raising and protruding your jaw.

Repeat fifteen to twenty times.

FACE STRETCHES

Rubber-mouth stretches *(top right)*

Open your mouth as wide as comfortably possible. Then make a variety of 'rubber mouth' expressions by moving your open mouth into different shapes.

Continue for fifteen to thirty seconds.

Neck stretch

Extend the long strap muscles in the sides of your neck by slowly turning your head first to one side, so you look as far over that shoulder as possible, then to the other. (*Caution*: stop if you feel dizzy or faint.)

Repeat five to ten times to each side.

Anti-frown stretches

See *Relaxing vertical lines* and *Relaxing horizontal lines* on page 152.

FACE 'WEIGHT' TRAINING

Mouth 'weight training'

Open your mouth into an 'O'. Rest the tips of your your thumb and forefinger inside your top and bottom lips, with their pads a centimetre apart. Try for ten to fifteen seconds to force your thumb and finger together with your lips, but prevent this with the strength of your thumb and finger.

Repeat once or twice.

Do the exercise again with the tips of your thumb and forefinger inside the corners of your lips instead.

Cheek 'weight training'
(centre right)

Either sit at a table or desk, or stand by the kitchen work-surface. Put your elbows on the surface and cup your head with your hands so the fleshy parts of your cheeks rest on the 'heels' of your hands, your

fingers on your temples and, most important, your hands take the weight of your head. If this doesn't happen, adust your position, perhaps by raising the height of your chair with a cushion. Smile, and feel your cheek muscles tighten against the heels of your hands; if you can't feel this, adjust the position of your hands.

Repeat twenty times.

Upper-eyelid 'weight training' *(bottom right)*

Look down behind closed eyes. Put a fingertip in the centre of each upper eyelid, just above the lashes. Repeatedly try to open your eyes, keeping the lids closed with your fingertips. Continue for five seconds.

Repeat five to ten times.

> ### Tip
>
> Doing a workout for your facial muscles makes an excellent way of helping to counteract any tension held there when you're feeling especially stressed.

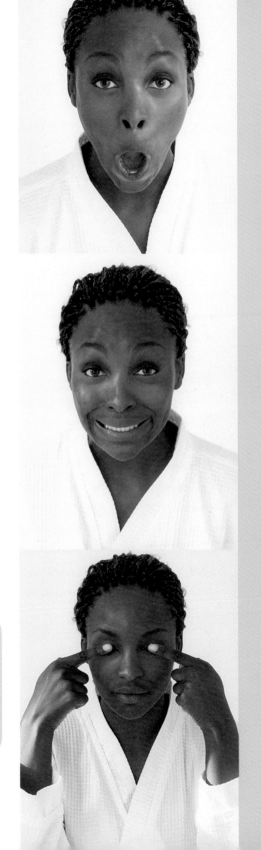

breathing for beauty

Each one of us needs to get enough good clean fresh air to keep our body fit and healthy, and our skin glowing, smooth and supple. But if your breathing rate is too fast or too slow, or if the air you breathe is polluted or stale, the levels of carbon dioxide and oxygen in your blood may stray outside their normal healthy ranges.

This disturbs the blood's acidity level (which is known to scientists as its 'pH'). This, in turn, means our body doesn't get enough oxygen, so we feel less fit and alert; we're more likely to succumb to fatigue, weakness and illness, and our complexion becomes tired-looking, dull and generally jaded.

The brain and kidneys usually work together to stop this happening. The brain can alter our breathing rate; the kidneys can adjust our blood's acidity level by changing the composition of the urine; and several other of the body's complex internal balancing mechanisms (called 'buffering systems') also help to regulate acidity. But if our acidity level is already too high or too low, this may not be good enough, and our skin may then get less oxygen that it needs. This can happen if you eat a lot of acid-forming foods, such as meat, eggs, and foods made with sugar or white flour. It can also happen if you're breathing rapidly because you are stressed, if your circulation is poor, or if you have a long-term heart, lung or kidney disease.

Continued poor oxygenation could make you more prone to premature wrinkling and thinning of the skin, and to asthma, depression, obesity, chronic fatigue syndrome (previously known as myalgic encephalomyelitis, or ME), and even certain cancers.

As well as oxygen, healthy skin needs enough water and heat, and not too much in the way of exposure to positive ions (minute airborne electrically charged particles that are attracted from the air to the skin), or other potentially harmful airborne substances, such as the particles and gases in cigarette smoke.

GOOD CIRCULATION

Your heart and arteries must be fit and healthy if they are to be capable of pumping and carrying enough oxygen to the skin cells and removing enough carbon dioxide from them. Chapters 3, 4 and 5 (on eating, exercising and de-stressing) will help you keep your whole cardiovascular system in good condition.

CLEAN AIR

Breathing dirty air ages skin prematurely because it is likely to be low in oxygen and because inhaled pollutants create potentially damaging substances in the skin called free radicals. One of the worst culprits is carbon monoxide, present in vehicle-exhaust emissions and fumes from poorly combusted household gas in faulty ovens and heating appliances. Even small quantities of carbon monoxide can prevent enough oxygen reaching skin cells. Another common air pollutant is cigarette smoke (also a source of carbon monoxide), which can be a problem for those who smoke and for those who inhale other people's smoke. Both smoking and passive smoking are bad news for the skin in many ways (see page 75).

TIPS FOR PROTECTING YOUR SKIN

- Stop smoking or, at least, cut down (see *Quit*, page 157).
- Ask smokers to stop or go elsewhere; open windows; or go elsewhere yourself.
- Use your car less, reduce exhaust emissions with regular servicing, and avoid speeding or over-revving.
- Support political clean-air initiatives.
- Move somewhere less polluted, if possible.
- Exercise indoors when pollution is bad.
- Take 500–1000mg of vitamin C each day; three hours in polluted air halves the amount of vitamin C in your skin.
- Reduce carbon monoxide and carbon dioxide indoors by growing ivies, spider plants, peace lilies, chrysanthemums, rubber plants, coconut palms, weeping figs, gerberas, dracaenas, and Boston ferns, all of which absorb small amounts of these gases.
- Don't even think about using commercially produced 'air fresheners'. They just disguise smells.

FRESH AIR

Breathing stale air can trigger 'air hunger', with yawning, fatigue and poor concentration; if you spend much time in stuffy places, your skin may age faster.

HUMIDITY, TEMPERATURE AND POSITIVE IONS

Many people work in a dry environment with only 25 percent humidity instead of the recommended 40–50 percent. Dry air evaporates water from the lungs, which in turn dehydrates the skin, making it dull and lined and reducing its resilience.

Counteract this by drinking plenty and humidifying the air with bowls of water over radiators and with flowers or well-watered pot plants. However, if you use well-watered pot plants as a way of increasing the air humidity at home or at work, make sure you don't let the soil in the pots become stale, because stale, moist soil encourages the growth of microscopic organisms called moulds. Some of these are known to encourage asthma and other lung disease.

Moist air contains fewer dustborne positive ions to irritate the skin. Positive ions are electrically charged particles that are generated by electro-magnetic fields around electrical appliances such as computer screens. They are found in higher concentrations in hot, dry air, and because of their electrostatic charge, they are attracted to the moistness of the facial skin. The problem with positive ions on the skin is that it can make the skin irritated, red and patchy. To beat this problem: increase the humidity level of the air in the room (see above); splash your face with water every two hours, wash away positive ions; and invest in an ionizer, a small electronic gadget that generates a stream of negatively charged ions to neutralize the positive ones.

AVOID TOO MUCH ACID-FORMING FOOD

Eating meat, fish, dairy products, eggs, white flour, nuts, beans and sugar makes blood more acidic. Normally this doesn't matter. But if you also breathe inappropriately, or breathe stale or polluted air, your body could become overloaded with acid. This is because while the brain copes with slightly raised acidity by encouraging faster breathing, this protective action stops when the body becomes too acidic. You then breathe out less carbon dioxide and inhale and use less oxygen, so your skin suffers.

breathe well

Breathing well usually comes naturally. But it's possible, particularly when stressed, to find yourself taking very shallow breaths. To get more air, you then breathe too fast (hyperventilate).

This means you exhale too much carbon dioxide. This, in turn, lowers the blood's acidity and constricts tiny arteries, which makes it hard for skin, nerve and muscle cells to get enough oxygen. Rapid breathing also makes the brain suspect danger, so it raises the body's adrenaline level. This creates a feeling of anxiety that is bad for the skin as explained in the next chapter. Breathing at the appropriate rate and depth for what you are doing is good for the skin. The average healthy person takes thirteen to seventeen breaths a minute at rest. Some yoga therapists claim as few as eleven to twelve is better. You can measure your rate by counting the number of whole breaths you take in one minute.

If your breathing tends to be shallow, be sure to take some daily exercise. This encourages deeper, slower breathing by reminding you how it feels to fill your lungs. The same goes for taking occasional deep breaths. When you take a deep breath, help your lungs expand fully by stretching your arms out sideways, or by 'breathing from your tummy', allowing it to protrude each time you inhale.

BREAK THE HABIT OF RAPID, SHALLOW BREATHING

When overly high stress levels continue, it's easy to fall into the habit of rapid, shallow breathing. And with more and more people complaining of a high stress level, increasing numbers are also breathing this way as a matter of course. These three

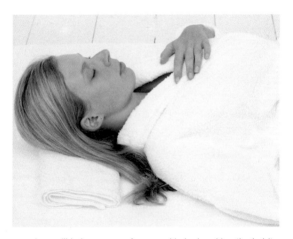

exercises will help you care for your skin by breaking the habit of rapid, shallow breathing.

Take a break

Sit in a chair with your feet flat on the floor, or lie on your back on the floor. Put one hand on your chest, the other on your tummy, and take slow, deep, relaxing breaths 'into your tummy' for up to ten minutes. Allow thoughts and images to pass through your mind without dwelling on them.

A quick fix

1 Stand with your feet hip-width apart and your knees 'unlocked'. With one loose, sweeping movement, take a slow, deep breath in while at the same time raising your arms straight out in front and then up above your head.

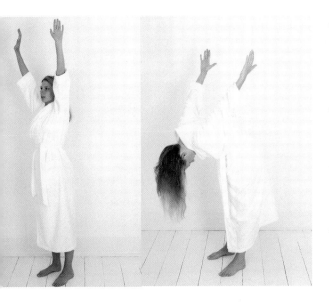

<big>1</big> Put the forefinger and middle finger of your left hand on the bridge of your nose. Breathe out through both nostrils.

<big>2</big> Now put your thumb over the side of your left nostril to close it and inhale through your right nostril.

<big>3</big> Close your right nostril with your fourth finger, lift your thumb off the left nostril and breathe out.

<big>4</big> Pause. Then, leaving your finger in place, inhale through your left nostril.

<big>5</big> Now close the left nostril with your thumb and breathe out through the right one.

Repeat the cycle five times and do the exercise each day while trying to break a rapid-shallow-breathing habit.

<big>2</big> Hold your breath and keep your arms in that position, for four or five seconds.

<big>3</big> Swing your arms down while breathing out and bending your back, hips and knees. Continue the movement so your arms swing behind you, letting your knees straighten a little.

<big>4</big> With one loose, sweeping movement, take a slow, deep breath and swing your arms back down towards the floor, then out in front and up above your head. Your knees should bend as your arms swing down and straighten on the upswing.

Repeat steps 2, 3 and 4 up to five times and do the whole exercise once or twice a day.

Alternate-nostril breathing

Like any slow, deep nasal breathing, this slows the heart rate, lowers blood pressure and reduces levels of stress. Do it at any time, sitting comfortably and breathing rhythmically and slowly.

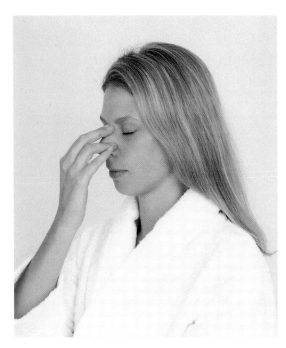

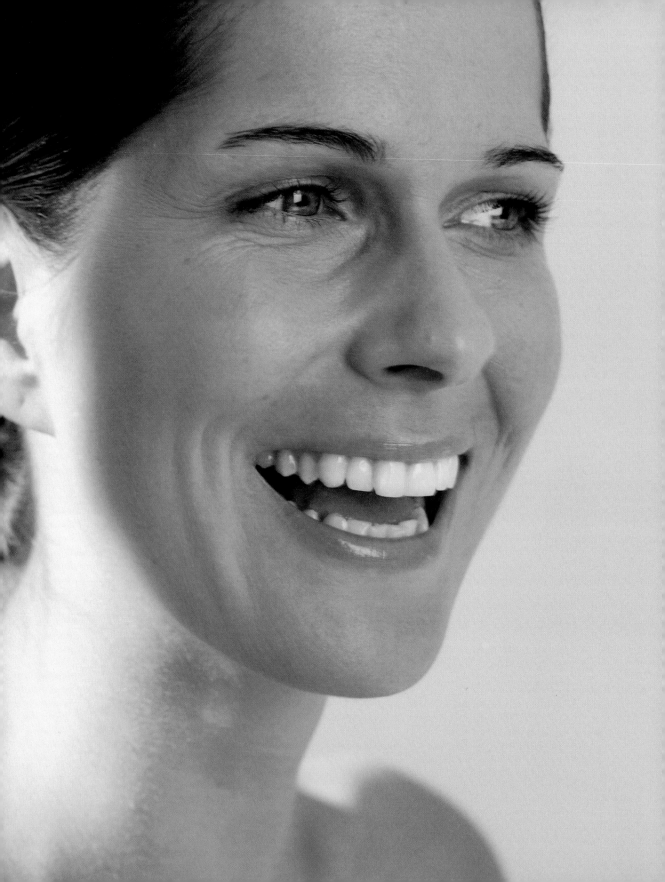

de-stressing

Stress and the skin are closely related. If we feel stressed for long, our skin will look older than its years, as well as tight, blotchy and less than its best. Prolonged stress disturbs our physical and mental well-being, and disrupting either can upset the well-being of the skin's blood supply, nerves and muscles.

Normally the body copes well with the various sorts of physical or mental stimulation we get every day; indeed, we need these if we are to stay alive and healthy. But any uncomfortable stimulus – such as illness, shock, emotional unease, or too much heat or cold – is stressful. This is where the importance of effective stress management comes in.

The key to managing stress lies in being able to recognise when you are stressed. You can then deal wisely with it and with your reactions to it.

the value of stress

Surprising as it may seem, stress can benefit our mental well-being – and that of our face too. The stresses we encounter add interest and excitement to life and, managed wisely, also help us know ourselves better.

With severe stress, all you may be able to hope for is to stick in there and survive. But even then some people discover something unexpected but important. Like metal tempered in a fire, they emerge stronger and brighter. The experience gives them new perspectives. Life takes on a different meaning and their values, attitudes and beliefs become refined. The heaviness of the stress paradoxically leads to a degree of enlightenment. Some people then find that when the next major stress arrives, they can, in a sense, welcome it. They know it will pass and they also know that it could eventually enrich them.

Stress raises the blood levels of cortisol, adrenaline and noradrenaline. These hormones prepare the body to produce extra energy so it is physically and mentally able to respond by 'fight or flight'. Both these use up the extra hormones. If you 'freeze' by doing nothing, or 'flow' with the stress by managing it effectively, the extra hormones gradually dissipate – unless, that is, your state of stress remains or keeps recurring.

WHEN STRESS GETS TOO MUCH

An episode of severe stress is one problem. Feeling continuously or repeatedly stressed is quite another. This may result from continuing or repeated problems, or may mean your body has become so used to being stressed that even when the actual stresses are over, it continues to react as if they were still there.

All is well if you lower your high stress-hormone levels by managing your stressed state effectively. If you don't, chronically high levels of stress hormones interfere with sleep, which is bad news for the skin because it is during the sleeping hours that new skin cells grow. What's more, feeling constantly stressed encourages frowning and a tight, 'drawn' face with dull eyes.

The continuous stimulation from high levels of cortisol during unrelieved stress eventually exhausts the body's supply of dihydroepiandrostenone (DHEA), the substance from which cortisol is made. The cortisol level then falls, which can trigger exhaustion and an inability to cope. Thiis s the condition that is popularly called a 'nervous breakdown'.

Continuing unrelieved stress lowers immunity, so encouraging skin infections and auto-immune problems affecting the skin (in which immune cells turn against the very cells they would normally protect). Raised stress-hormone levels also narrow arteries and therefore encourage poor circulation. They do this by making artery-wall muscles tense and encouraging fatty deposits of atheroma to block arteries. This is why your skin looks dull and lifeless when you feel stressed. Poor circulation also encourages the skin to age prematurely.

Another problem from constantly raised stress-hormone levels is that diabetes is more likely. A raised level of stress hormones increases the blood-sugar level. This triggers the pancreas (a gland behind the stomach) to produce more insulin so as to use and store this excess sugar. But an overstimulated pancreas may eventually wear out, leading to diabetes, with a lack of insulin and a consequent – and potentially dangerous – rise in blood sugar and disturbance in blood fats. This encourages heart disease which, in turn, leads to poor circulation.

The signs of stress

Stresses come in all sorts of guises and it's important to develop a strategy for recognising your body's own particular signs of stress.

RECOGNISING THE SIGNS OF STRESS

The signs of stress are surprisingly varied from one person to another, but tend to be similar in any one individual. They include:

- stiff, aching, tense muscles
- poor sleep
- headaches
- anxiety
- sweating and shaking
- depression
- indigestion
- tiredness
- frequent illness through infection
- hyperventilation.

Tests may reveal high blood pressure and a high cholesterol level too. Stress may also trigger potentially harmful behaviours such as:

- comfort eating
- other eating disorders
- smoking
- gambling/risk-taking
- alcohol binges or dependency
- over-work
- repeated unrewarding relationships
- disinterest in sex
- apathy
- aggressive, passive or passive-aggressive (victim-like) behaviour.

ways of beating stress

It's good to recognize your response to stress because you can then use one or more stress-management techniques to lower your stress-hormone levels and protect yourself and your skin. Stress-management strategies come in many guises. The trick is to know what to choose and when you need to try something different.

Use quick fixes when time is short but be sure to incorporate long-term solutions into your daily life. The combination will work wonders for you and your skin.

QUICK FIXES

Choose from these quick fixes when stressed.

Take action

Stress hormones give you energy to be assertive if necessary. This means making your needs clear without hurting the other person or putting them down. If you have to bottle up stress-induced energy, deal with it later. If being aggressive or running away seem necessary, your stress will probably give you plenty of energy (though some people find the opposite is true).

Get moving

Exercising enough to boost your heart rate and make you warmer 'burns' up surplus stress hormones.

Go outside

Get some daylight on your skin to boost your level of oestrogen, and of vitamin D which is now thought to raise the level of a 'feel-good' chemical called serotonin.

Take a break

Take a few minutes off to relax, have a nap, or simply turn off, by leafing through a magazine or going outside for a stroll. It is important always to have a lunchtime break too. This can dissipate stress hormones and help put problems and challenges into perspective.

Take a breather

Take some slow, deep breaths for two minutes every hour and, as you do this, try to let all the excess nervous tension flow from you.

Restore the inner person

Coffee, tea and cola are stimulants, so some people prefer water or herb tea when stressed. But while guzzling lots of tea and coffee will probably make stress worse, an occasional cup can be comforting. Alcohol tends to magnify your current mood. However, as long as a tipple does not take you over recommended limits (14 units a week for non-pregnant women, 21 for men), it can be a pleasant way of unwinding.

Opt for a carbohydrate-based snack to boost serotonin. Bread, bananas, potatoes and dates are good choices. And stock up on foods rich in vitamin C (see page 47).

Prioritize tasks, plan your time and delegate

List tasks according to what you have to achieve first. Jot down how long you think each will realistically take. Delegate anything you can. Then, if necessary, accept that you will have to do some tasks another day.

Talk it over

It is nearly always true that a problem shared is a problem halved.

Laugh

Find something, anything, to laugh at. If you can't, laugh at nothing. This boosts your level of 'feel-good' endorphins.

Have a change

In your work, social or domestic life, remember that a change is often as good as a rest.

Stretch

Relax a tense back and shoulders with this lovely stretch.

1 Lie flat on your back on the floor, arms relaxed and loosely clasped hands resting low on your abdomen.

2 Slowly breathe in and raise your arms, hands still joined and elbows straight, above your head.

3 Now slowly breathe out while lowering your arms until they come to rest as far as possible behind your head on the floor.

4 Pause for a few seconds without breathing to feel the stretch.

5 Reverse the exercise by breathing in as you return your hands to the vertical, and out as you lower them to your abdomen. Press your hands gently into your abdomen.

Repeat the whole cycle five or six times.

Have a scented bath

Run the water, add five or six drops of lavender, rose or neroli oil and soak for twenty minutes. After, drying, scoop up some floating oil and rub it gently into your forehead.

Have sex (with someone else or on your own)

Making time for this age-old pleasure is an excellent way of de-stressing yourself.

Think of something that makes you happy

Focus your mind for a few minutes on someone or something you love.

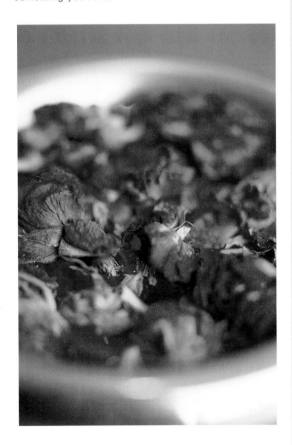

LONG-TERM SOLUTIONS

It isn't desirable, sensible or even possible to clear every source of stress from your life. So the answer is to manage it and your reaction to it effectively. Quick fixes are one way. Long-term solutions are another. The most important of these is to give your lifestyle a makeover by assessing – or re-assessing – how you could rid yourself of unnecessary stresses and alter your response so as to make yourself more stress-proof.

Balance

Discover what proportion of your life you spend sleeping, working, eating and drinking, doing everyday tasks, enjoying meaningful relationships, relaxing and meditating (or praying). It helps to list these categories for each day of the week and work out roughly how much time you spend on each. There is no right or wrong, but you may find you want to rebalance your day. If this means changing your work or domestic life, or forging better relationships, talk it over with a trusted person if necessary, and start putting the changes in place.

Management

If you are to manage stress effectively, you need to learn to be a good manager. Good managers in any sphere take enough quiet time to assess what is going on and to work out what is needed to help things happen more smoothly and fruitfully. So programme some management time into each day and use it to be observant and creative. Imagine, for example, that you are a helicopter and can look down at what's going on in your domestic or working life. You are more important than the biggest company in the world and

there is no reason why you shouldn't benefit from the very skills that are being taught to managers of innumerable companies and other organisations every day.

Exercise

This is one of the most important ways of stress-proofing yourself. It helps keep every part of your body, including your skin, in good condition. It entails taking at least half an hour of exercise on at least five days of the week. (Chapter 4 outlines what to choose.) Ironically, stress is the biggest enemy of regular exercise, because it's so easy to find reasons for putting off exercising when you are busy, upset or anxious. So when you least want to exercise is the very time it is most important for your health and well-being. Try overcoming this hurdle by using any reluctance to exercise as a trigger for making sure you get moving. Involving someone else or being part of a group helps with this.

Food

Eating well (see Chapter 3) provides you with the nutrients you need for you and your body to cope well with stress. Choose a healthy balance of food to help protect your arteries, keep your nerves and muscles working well and encourage glowing, vital skin. Certain foods can be particularly helpful in keeping you feeling calm and capable of coping when you are going through a stressful time. And it's worth noting that a longterm lack of the nutrients listed below can actually encourage feelings of anxiety. These nutrients, together with the main foods that are particularly rich in them, include:

- complex carbohydrates such as those in wholegrain foods, root vegetables, beans, peas and bananas

- the B vitamin called niacin, found in milk, fish, meat, nuts, mushrooms, dates and seeds
- vitamin E, found in dairy food, eggs, fish, meat, wholegrain foods, beans, nuts, green leafy vegetables, seeds, and sprouted seeds
- calcium, found in dairy food, eggs, wholegrain foods, beans, nuts, green leafy vegetables, root vegetables, dates and seeds
- magnesium, found in fish, meat, wholegrain foods, beans, nuts, green leafy vegetables, mushrooms and seeds

Breathing

Don't forget to assess your breathing pattern. Continued stress encourages the habit of hyperventilation (see page 64) which, in turn, can make the body less resilient to the effects of stress. Unfortunately, it is all too easy to let this go unnoticed.

Pain relief

Medical problems that cause long-term pain are a potent source of stress. However, a lot is known nowadays about ways of relieving this sort of pain. It makes every sense to manage chronic pain by consulting your doctor and asking for a referral to a pain specialist if necessary.

Listening and being listened to

Many a promising relationship flounders because neither person knows how to listen properly. Skilful listening enables each person to feel heard and understood. It involves three steps. The first is to put your own feelings temporarily to one side. The second is to identify your partner's main emotions. And the third is to let them know you have attempted to do this (even if you are wrong) by feeding back with a comment such as, 'It sounds as if you're feeling scared/angry/worried.' That really is all it takes!

Listening to yourself

What many people don't take on board, though, is the huge help it can be – especially during times of particular stress – to know how to listen to yourself. To do this, you need to use exactly the same three stages of listening skills outlined above.

First, wait until your mind feels calm enough to 'listen' – or take note – of the emotions you are experiencing. Second, give a name to your main emotion, or emotions. And, third, test whether you're right by thinking about whether you really are, for example, angry, scared, or even desperate.

Listening to yourself is an extremely useful habit, because it helps prevent unrecognized emotions from overwhelming you. Just knowing you have recognized and acknowledged difficult emotions reduces their power to make you stressed. It prevents unrecognized and unacknowledged emotions in your unconscious mind from controlling your behaviour and encouraging stress-related habits such as comfort eating, smoking or drinking too much, taking illegal drugs, and having affairs in a supposedly one-to-one relationship. So it gives you more control over the way you live your life. And it lets you progress to find other ways of managing what is going on in your life.

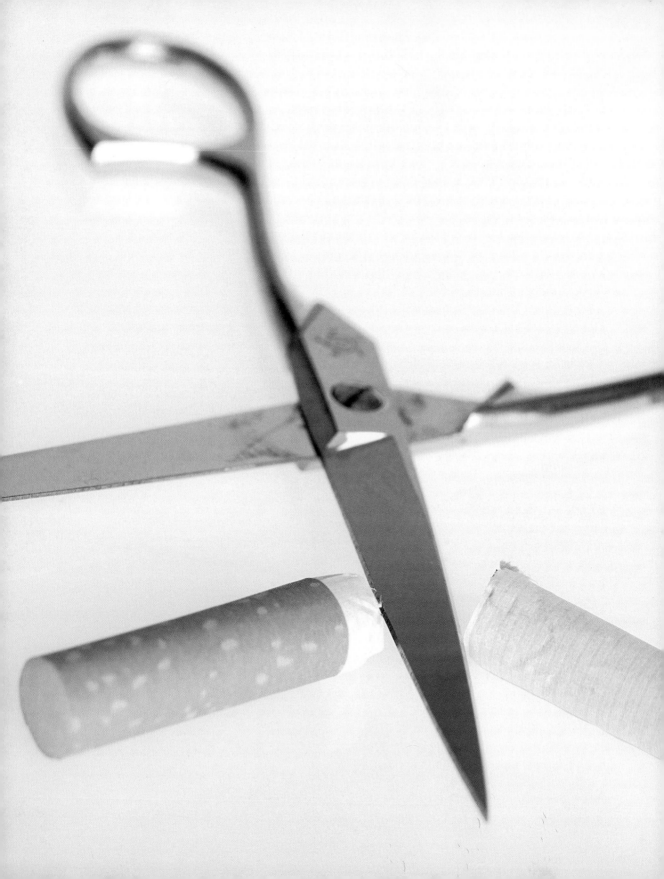

healing unwanted habits

Smoking and drinking are two of the many habits that can do your skin a lot of harm.

SMOKING

Women who smoke are three times as likely as non-smokers to have lined, wrinkled, grey, leathery, prematurely aged skin – or a 'cigarette face'. At the age of forty, a heavy smoker's skin is like that of a sixty-year-old non-smoker. Passive smoking – breathing other people's smoke – is bad for skin too. Smoking and passive smoking are the skin's enemies for the following reasons.

- Carbon monoxide inhaled in reduces the skin's oxygen supply.
- Many of the 4000 or so other toxins in each puff of smoke encourage the formation of many billions of free radicals at a time. These diminish the skin's oxygen supply by encouraging fatty atheroma to clog up arteries.
- Smoking twenty cigarettes a day restricts your skin's oxygen supply for most of the day. Over the years this makes skin lined, thin and generally 'kippered'.
- Your body uses 25mg of vitamin C to counteract the free radicals formed by each cigarette; this means that smokers go short of this skin-friendly antioxidant vitamin.
- Chemicals from inhaled smoke raise stress-hormone levels; adversely affect collagen and elastin, connective tissue proteins necessary for skin 'bounce' and strength; and thin the skin by 25–40 percent, so encouraging wrinkles and lowering the body's oestrogen level, which in women encourages an early menopause.
- Cadmium in cigarette smoke makes skin dry and scaly.
- The heat of a burning cigarette held near the face, together with some of the numerous harmful substances in its smoke, can directly damage skin.
- Smoking encourages chest infections, heart disease, skin cancer and auto-immune diseases.
- Smoking twenty cigarettes a day makes excess facial hair 50 percent more likely.

STOPPING SMOKING

Smokers who cannot – or do not want to – stop or cut down can help protect their skin by inhaling as little as possible, holding the cigarette well away from their face, and blowing exhaled air far away. Smokers should also use good sun-protection; and eat plenty of foods rich in antioxidants such as beta-carotene, vitamins C and E and selenium.

DRINKING

The habit of drinking in excess can be bad for the skin in many ways. It can:

- dehydrate the skin by flushing increased volumes of water from the body in the urine
- lead to poor circulation in the skin
- cause stress, which indirectly harms the skin by further reducing its circulation
- encourage accidents
- raise your risk of many illnesses, several of which – including high blood pressure, liver damage, depression, heart disease and alcohol addiction – have negative effects on the skin
- encourage obesity and malnourishment, because alcohol is high in calories and low in nutrients and dampens the appetite for more nutritious foods.

SEARCHING FOR NEW STRATEGIES

If stress underlies your smoking or drinking, search for other ways of managing it that will harm neither you nor your skin. First, though, try to understand why you turn to smoking or drinking. This could, for example, be because you find that it soothes anxiety or other difficult feelings; makes you feel clearer-headed, more confident and in control, or too sleepy to dwell on problems; helps you communicate and feel part of the crowd; or simply makes you feel good. If you – or your nearest and dearest – are really concerned, how about seeking help from a counsellor or therapist?

An effective stress-management strategy is successful and lasting. This means it must offer similar benefits to those from smoking or drinking, or, preferably, better ones. If it doesn't, your yearning for the comfort and familiarity of your old habit may easily sabotage it.

Any new strategy to combat harmful habits will feel odd, but practice will soon make it familiar. If it doesn't help, try something else, getting any help you need from your doctor, a counsellor or a self-help group. Finally, remember that relapsing into your old habit of drinking or smoking doesn't mean you are a failure. Just try again. Many roads to success are paved with 'failures'.

SLEEPING BETTER

A good night's sleep is worth its weight in gold to you and your face. You wake up feeling brighter and better able to meet challenges. And it's during unbroken sleep that most skin-cell regeneration and healing occurs. However, so many things affect the quality and quantity of sleep that sleep problems are common. So how can you improve your chances of dropping off and sleeping well? Hopefully, the following tips will help.

- Check that your bed feels really comfortable; your pillow is adjusted to give your neck and head the right support when you are lying on your back or side; and your bed-covers are not too hot, cold, heavy or otherwise uncomfortable.
- Invest in some closely fitting earplugs if your partner's snoring, road din, or other external noise keeps you awake. Such earplugs can reduce the sound level by up to 20 decibels.
- Avoid cocoa, as well as cola, coffee and tea (unless decaffeinated) after 4pm, as their caffeine can be a potent stimulant.

- Take half-an-hour's daily exercise, but do this no later than five or six hours before bedtime, because otherwise you may find its after-effects stimulating instead of relaxing.

- Say 'no' to an evening nap, however tempting this may be at the time, as this could keep you awake for several hours when you should ideally be getting a long, uninterrupted run of sleep.

- Have your last meal early, and keep later snacks small, light, carbohydrate-rich and cheese-free.

- Drink soothing vervain, lemon balm or hop tea instead of a milky or alcoholic nightcap. Milk lies on some people's tummy, and alcohol can be stimulating, especially if you already feel excited and full of energy.

- Encourage your mind to switch off by enjoying a warm pre-bedtime bath scented with a camomile teabag or a few drops of lavender oil.

- Experiment with the herbal remedies valerian or passiflora; the homeopathic remedy Coffea; or an amino-acid food supplement called 5-hydroxy tryptophan.

- Discuss effective problem and stress-management techniques with a friend or counsellor if worry – about work or money problems, for example – stops you sleeping.

- If you simply cannot sleep, relax with some soothing music.

- See your doctor if you've slept badly for over two weeks, and are exhausted, depressed, desperate, or unable to drive or cope with your job and family.

IMPROVING YOUR POSTURE

Your posture can readily affect your feelings, both physical and emotional, and your feelings, in turn, can readily affect the way you look.

Habitual poor posture encourages an aching back and shoulders, a stiff neck, a tight scalp, a tense jaw, and shallow breathing. These encourage depression, dejection, anxiety and stress, as well as tension of face and body muscles, which may make posture even worse.

However, sometimes it's the other way round, and depression, oppression, tension, anxiety, anger or muscle tension cause poor posture. A person may feel they have the cares of the world on their shoulders, but without enough support. Other people may be 'on their back', and life seems too much to bear. They suffer from a low self-esteem and hold themselves as if trying to disappear. Indeed, holding feelings 'in the body' like this is relatively common.

Whatever the cause, deal with poor posture by finding a way of reminding yourself at intervals throughout the day to hold yourself better. Aim to stand with your head well balanced over your spine and your shoulders back, so your neck and shoulder muscles don't work overtime. Holding yourself erect can be like smiling. If you smile when feeling low, your mood often lifts. Likewise, if you straighten up when feeling low, you may feel better and brighter in mind and body.

Get to the root of any emotional distress and learn to manage it more effectively. And sort out any physical cause of poor posture, such as carrying a heavy weight (perhaps a bag or a child) on one side; sitting or working in an uncomfortable position; or wearing high heels for too long. If necessary, an Alexander technique teacher can help you become more aware of your balance, posture and movement.

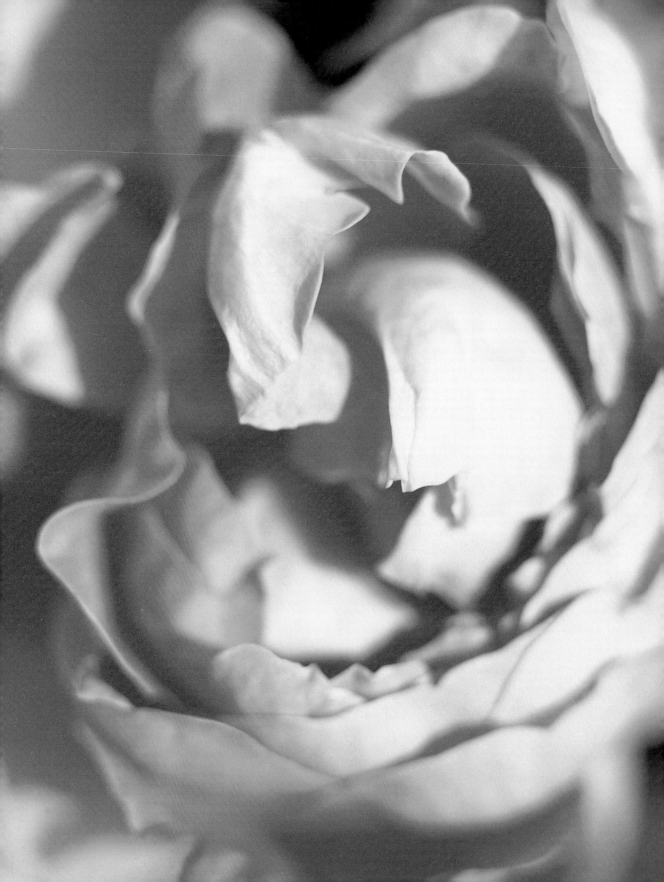

finding an
inner radiance

Some people radiate a beauty that has nothing to do with the shape of their face, the quality of their skin or the flattery of their make-up. They look lovely because their face reveals an inner beauty that shines through as clearly as if their skin were transparent. We catch glimpses of such attributes as an unconditional love for others, an acceptance of themselves and an enthusiasm for everyday life and the challenges it brings. We sometimes feel almost as if we are looking into their heart, mind and soul. And we like what we see.

Such beauty makes these individuals very attractive, however quirky, ordinary or even ugly their face may be. What is more, this beauty can act as a shining beacon that lights the road they are taking through life and provides a source of inspiration and encouragement to others.

outer beauty

Compared with the benefits of inner beauty, those of a surgical facelift pale into insignificance. The good news is that each one of us can cultivate our inner beauty. As it grows you will find it will increasingly light your path through life too. We will look now at a few ideas for living your life in a way that makes the most of your personality, opportunities and gifts; allows you to enjoy, love and encourage yourself and those around you; and enables you to explore and satisfy your deepest yearnings.

They say that beauty is in the eye of the beholder, meaning we can perceive someone as being beautiful if we recognise their inner beauty, love them or have some other intimate connection with them. But when it comes to what constitutes actual physical – or 'outer' – beauty, there is remarkable agreement. Research psychologists have found that our appreciation of outer beauty is based on our unconscious recognition of certain 'ideal' facial proportions (such as widely spaced, big eyes, or high cheekbones) that have cultural, temporal, racial and gender-specific associations with beauty.

Outer beauty often has a fascinating effect on other people's responses.

THE PHYSICALLY BEAUTIFUL FACE

There is no doubting the pleasure that the looks of a physically beautiful woman can give to others (and also, hopefully, to herself). The positive way that most people respond is bound to colour her experience of life and her expectations of relationships, both current and future. Superficially, at least, all this must make life somewhat easier for her in certain ways.

But we must not forget that this kind of obvious beauty can make some other individuals jealous, critical or spiteful, for reasons that have nothing to do with the woman as an individual or, indeed, with any comparison they may make with their own looks. Her appearance may trigger echoes from previous difficult and unresolved situations they have experienced. It may also underline their own lack of self-esteem in an uncomfortable way. Having said this, though, it's also true that people may respond negatively to a physically beautiful woman in response to her behaviour or personality.

Whether other people's reactions to a beautiful woman are positive or negative, it isn'tt always easy to know if this is because of her looks, her behaviour or her personality. Yet what we all really want is to be loved for who we are on the inside. So sometimes being physically beautiful can be extremely confusing.

THE ORDINARY FACE

In contrast, the woman with an ordinary face that doesn't stand out in a crowd does not experience such heightened and contrasting reactions. People who react positively to her are much more likely to do so because they like her personality, sense of humour or inner beauty, or because they are acting with unconditional human warmth. So from that point of view things are more predictable.

WHAT ABOUT MEN AND THIER LOOKS?

For many decades in the twentieth century, society put the importance of men's looks on the back burner. But in the last ten years we've seen a rapidly growing interest in male 'beauty'. You have only to look at men's magazines, clothes shops and grooming products to see this is so.

Male beauty, good looks or handsomeness may or may not coexist with attractiveness and sex appeal. And the dilemmas, challenges and benefits for a good-looking man are similar in many ways to those experienced by a beautiful woman.

SELF-ESTEEM

You might think positive reactions to physical beauty would boost an individual's self-esteem. But this is likely only if they have little sense of self-worth. Self-esteem based on other people's valuation of your looks has little real or lasting value. It feels precarious – and it is. If they love you this conditionally, you realize they could stop loving you one day. While you may thrive on their praise and admiration, these do not make the 'real you' feel lovely and loveable, so they are not truly nourishing.

Feeling loved and valued

It is the experience of being loved and valued for your individuality, personality and potential that nourishes the real you and makes you feel truly loveable and valuable. Your self-esteem now becomes a real, lasting and solid base for life. It can then contribute to your inner beauty. And the wonderful bonus is that it enables you to love and value others for themselves, without needing anything in return.

Relationships

All sorts of relationships can encourage the development of healthy self-esteem, including those with parents, friends, teachers, a partner, colleagues, an employer, a counsellor, a minister and, through their books, with authors. Many people say their relationship with God is pivotal too.

Behaviour

Having a healthy self-esteem allows you to distinguish between your behaviour and the 'real you'. You may sometimes dislike your behaviour or that of others, but you will not confuse it with the whole person. You know behaviour can be changed. You also know this is more likely if a person has experienced being – and feeling – loved, and so feels loveable and therefore has a sense of self-worth. This gives them the 'oomph' they need to 'become what they could be', rather than remain as they are. And, as we shall see, it can add to their inner beauty.

the effect of your inner life on your looks

Most people agree that a face made luminous and lovely by inner beauty is just as attractive as one that is beautiful only on the outside, if not more so.

Inner beauty shows in such things as bright, lively eyes and a warm smile. You feel such a person likes you. A physically beautiful person who also has inner beauty may be amazingly lovely, but without inner beauty they may be much less attractive than they have the potential to be. An uncomfortable inner life can spoil their overall beauty by encouraging either an impassive mask-like expression, or frowning, dull eyes and a hard-set jaw.

Similarly, the face of an ordinary-looking or even an ugly person who is rich in inner beauty may light up with loveliness. But with a barren inner life they too are less attractive.

The Greek philosopher Plato debated the concepts of beauty, truth and justice, and it's interesting to consider these in terms of the face. While the world may judge outer good looks as being the only 'beauty', the 'truth' of the presence or absence of inner beauty soon becomes apparent. And though some people inherit lovelier looks than others, the existence or otherwise of inner beauty means that 'justice' – in other words, their attractiveness and worth as an individual – will prevail.

THE LANGUAGE OF THE FACE

Our expressions generally reveal our emotions and thoughts. They 'talk' on our behalf even when we are quiet. Sometimes, though, we don't let our face show what is going on inside ourselves, and sometimes it reveals emotions of which we are not consciously aware.

We all use some expressions more than others, and our face also has a certain basic look in repose. Over the decades our habitual expressions shape our face and form the lines and contours of our facial 'map'. This is the reason for the old warning, 'If the wind changes while you are sulking, you'll look sulky for ever.'

If you aren't familiar with your habitual expressions, ask someone who knows you well. Knowing could be good news, because you might want to work on changing them. Frowning frequently without realising it, for example, could lead to permanent lines that make you look far older than your age. Effective stress management could lighten and loosen your face enough to give it a real lift.

SEX APPEAL AND ATTRACTION

Both outer and inner beauty can contribute to a person's attractiveness and sex appeal. But outer beauty isn't a necessity. Many people deemed physically plain are enormously attractive, either sexually or in other ways. Something about the way they move their face, talk, listen, hold eye contact, groom themselves, laugh, think, believe or act transforms their appearance. And as we'll see, there are various ways of boosting inner beauty that can make an enormous difference to any one of us.

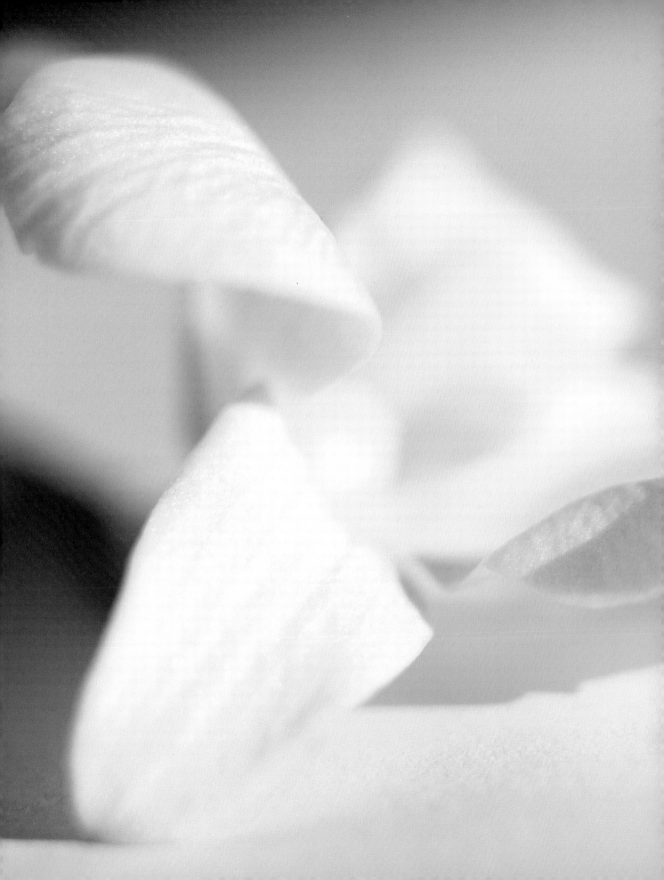

boosting your inner beauty

Time and effort spent boosting inner beauty is worth many facelifts. A person's inner beauty can comprise one or more of a very wide variety of gifts, arts and skills.

Use this list to decide what you want or need to develop further.

- Feeling loved and loveable (see *Self-esteem*, page 81).
- Making the most of opportunities.
- Living in the present, rather than in the past or future.
- Being enthusiastic and passionate.
- Focusing on good things rather than only on bad.
- Having a sense of humour.
- Encouraging yourself and others, especially when times are tough. Encouragement is a learnable skill in which you focus on what a person is endeavouring to do, as well as on what they have achieved. Simply describe what they are trying to do, or have done, and use listening skills to indicate your understanding of how this makes you feel.
- Welcoming the challenges that life brings rather than railing against them.
- Holding the hope that the difficulties you try to manage will ultimately have some benefit, even though this may not be apparent at the time.
- Learning to listen empathically to yourself, as well as to others. This involves identifying emotions (obvious and hidden) and using your acceptance of them – even of difficult ones such as anger, fear and despair – to understand yourself and others better.
- Arranging outlets for your creativity.
- Recognising your deepest yearnings and desires.

- Drawing strength from a relationship with God. You may, like most people in the world, choose to follow religious guidelines. New-age ideas can be helpful, but sometimes seem disconnected, shallow and unfulfilling when compared with the rich teachings, traditions and insights of – Christianity, Judaism, Islam and Buddhism.

POSTURE, LAUGHTER AND VOICE

Researchers say the way we use our body can have a profound influence on our state of mind. So try:

- If you feel low, making yourself laugh (even when you are not amused) can raise your level of endorphins (natural 'feel-good'substances in the blood) and help you feel more cheerful.
- If life is weighing heavily, a combination of straightening your back and shoulders, and holding your head up high, can make a world of difference.
- If you feel shy or afraid, breathing deeply, relaxing and adding more volume and resonance to your voice can work wonders.

So if you have been feeling and looking less than your bst, try adjusting your posture, having a laugh and making your voice strong as you sing a song or phone a friend.

Caution: These actions are no substitute for the proper treatment of clinical depression, for which you should initially consult your family doctor.

BEGINNING AND ENDING THE DAY

Another idea is to start and end the day with a quiet time. This could take the form of reflection, meditation or prayer. You could think about what the day may bring, the people you will meet and the things you will do. You could affirm a wish to do well by yourself and others, and consider any preparations you need to make. Some people ask God to be with them. And you could add the well-known request, 'Give us this day our daily bread', meaning that you would like to receive what you need – which might be the ability to deal with challenging circumstances, ask for help or recognise the 'teachers' that might come your way. Such teachers can come in unexpected guises: it is said that one always turns up when there is something we need to learn.

At the end of the day, make time to reflect on its events, your thoughts and feelings about the day, and what has been good in it, however small or trivial this may seem. Tiny specks of gold glister just as much as large nuggets and can quickly accumulate to enrich your life.

DOING WHAT MAKES YOU HAPPY

When you are finding life difficult, try this easy but revealing exercise. List up to ten things you love doing. Examples might include having a long, scented, relaxing bath, horse-riding, reading, seeing a friend, painting, listening to music, walking or learning something new. Now add four columns, headed: 'Every day', 'Once a week', 'Once a month' and 'Once a year'. Tick how often you do each of the things on your list.

Discussing your chart with a good friend, or with your partner, may suggest that the structure of your life needs changing to incorporate more of what enriches you.

VALUING YOUR LIFE STORY

Everyone's life has its ups and downs, but sometimes we go through a stretch which seems to have more than its fair share of problems. If you feel especially battered by life, it could be because difficult feelings are dammed up inside. In this case, making a graph of your life story could help you bring them out into the open and, perhaps, use them constructively.

1 Make the horizontal axis represent your age, starting from birth (or before, if big things happened to your mother or you when you were in the womb).

2 Enter along the horizontal axis the major things that have happened to you.

3 The vertical axis represents your emotional wellbeing; mark with a cross somewhere on this axis a value for each life event.

4 Join the crosses to produce a lifeline representing the ebb and flow of your emotional wellbeing.

5 Share this lifeline with your partner or a close friend.

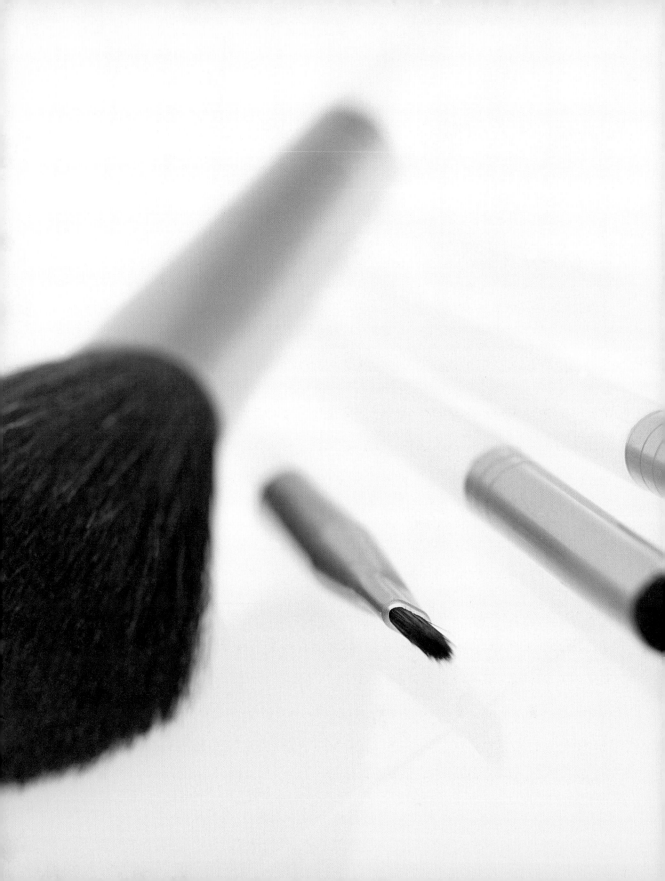

7 professional beauty secrets

There are few better ways of giving your face a natural lift than by looking good – and knowing you look good. Since time immemorial women of all ages, from young girls to white-haired great-grandmothers, have enjoyed beautifying themselves and each other. At various times in history men have taken more of an interest in enhancing their appearance too. In parallel, there have always been some people in every community who are especially interested and skilled in making other people look their best. Such people today work as make-up artists, hair stylists, beauticians, clothing and jewellery designers, wardrobe advisers and cosmetic–counter assistants.

We can learn a great deal from many of these professionals. And one of the most important things is to understand what sort of skin-care, make-up, hairstyle, jewellery and clothing best suits us as individuals.

time for yourself

Spend time looking after your skin, hair and clothes and you will not only feel good yourself, but you'll be doing those around you a favour too – for it's always much more pleasant to be with people who take care over their looks. And, in a sense, bothering to make yourself look good is a compliment to them. So however busy your life, programme in enough time each day to keep yourself looking your best.

All too often people make the mistake of following fashion with no regard to how it looks on them. Yet it's always a good idea to experiment with new looks and to see whether you, personally, are happy with them and whether they contribute to the enhancement of your appearance.

Many professional beauty basics and secrets, however, are unconnected with fashion and simply stand the test of time. So now we'll look at some tips to help you to care for your skin, to choose and apply your make-up, to do your hair and generally adorn your face, hair and body.

LOOKING SCRUFFY?

Almost everyone lets themselves look scruffy sometimes, but letting things slip for a large proportion of the time could mean that your unconscious mind is telling you and others something important about your state of mind. 'Acting out' distress and a lack of self-confidence in this way is surprisingly common. So cast your eye over your hair, skin, make-up, clothes and shoes, and if you think you look scruffy, ask yourself why, and if necessary, act now to work out why.

WHERE TO FIND BEAUTY BASICS AND SECRETS

The way to start making the most of your appearance is to use some of the basic discoveries made by the many women – and men – who have trodden this path before. There is no point in re-inventing the wheel! You can learn beauty basics and secrets from many sources, but the majority of women learn most from each other. Mothers pass them on to their daughters. Grandmothers, aunts, sisters and other female relations share the tips that they have learnt or discovered with each other. Friends copy each other and experiment together. You can pick up ideas from magazines, television, make-up and beauty counters, fashion shows and clothes shops. And you can even go on courses to help you master some of the tricks of the trade.

Once you have learnt the basic skills that can help you look good, you can then take advantage of some of the professional 'secrets' that can make such a big difference to every single one of of us. And then it is just a question of constantly experimenting to create your own individual look.

FASHION AND 'ANTI-FASHION'

If you wish, keep an eye on current fashions and take on board any that you like and that could give your overall appearance, including your make-up, hair and wardrobe, the look of the moment. Of course there is absolutely no need to be 'fashionable', and quite a few people purposefully refuse to have anything to do with fashion, preferring to adopt an 'anti-fashion' stance (which in some circles is fashionable in itself!). But while it certainly isn't clever to follow any fashion for the sake of it, especially if it doesn't suit you, being alert and interested in current trends can add zest and fun to life. And some commentators report that fashions in make-up, hair, and apparel in general reflect the Zeitgeist – the spirit of the age – remarkably accurately and in a variety of subtle and not-so-subtle ways. So by taking an interest in what is becoming popular, what is in and what is on its way out, or dead, you give yourself another window on the world.

FINDING YOUR OWN LOOK

Most of us like the idea of finding our own, individual look, one that marks us out as a person who knows who they are, where they are going, what suits them best and, perhaps, what they think is important. Of course, this doesn't mean we should always wear the same sorts of clothes or have our hair in the same style. So just how do we go about this task?

One way of helping yourself find your own style is by recognizing three things:

• What nature has given you.

• Your current looks.

• How you would like to look.

Whatever your basic appearance, you can learn to enhance it. And as you take the time and effort to make the most of your potential, you will find that your face begins to reflect your new-found source of animation. So quite apart from the flattering effect of your cosmetics, hairstyle, clothing and jewellery, your face will glow with the inner brightness that comes from looking after and maximizing your natural assets.

FINDING TIME TO LOOK AFTER YOURSELF

The hours and minutes often disappear most quickly when you most need them to look after yourself. One reason is that many of us are doing too much.

Women with children who work full-time are often particularly stressed, because they are more likely than their partner to shoulder the lion's share of domestic responsibilities. And when they are home, they want to cram in a lot of mothering. Working part-time isn't necessarily better, because it's tempting to think you should cope perfectly with everything, and to feel a failure when you can't. The workload is lightest for many mothers if they stay home. But this isn't always considered possible, because of financial reasons or lifestyle aspirations. And some women are so stressed by domesticity and child-care that going to work seems a positive relief.

However, whatever your domestic, childcare and working arrangements, it's vitally important to programme some time for yourself each day. Just half an hour can make all the difference. And you should see this as a right, not an indulgence. For no-one is well served if a lack of personal time means you let yourself go.

make-up

The biggest benefit from make-up is the fun of choosing and using it. Making up is the adult equivalent of playing with finger paints, with the added advantage of enhancing your face. So if you have never tried make-up, or have used the same cosmetics in the same way for years, browse around the cosmetics counters and give yourself a treat.

CHOOSING THE RIGHT COLOURS

If cream, russet, ochre, yellow, peach and orange tones in clothes light up your face and net you more compliments, go for make-up with hints of these warm colours. But if white, and bluish pinks and reds, do most for you, and anything with a yellowish tone makes your skin look dull, steer clear of any hint of yellow or orange.

A few simple cosmetic tricks can work wonders on the face.

EYES

Dark circles: Disguise with a stick concealer. Focus attention on the upper lid with a relatively dark shadow.

Droopy upper lids: Smooth some mid-taupe or grey cream eyeshadow over your lids; apply a thin line of dark, liquid eyeliner along the margin of the upper lids, then a powder shadow darker than the cream one over the liner and in each socket.

Puffy: Apply some chilled eye gel ten minutes before putting on your make-up. Use a matt shadow rather than a shimmering one. For under-eye puffiness, use a slightly darker concealer than normal.

Redness: Use a concealer or a green-toned or camouflage-type foundation.

Bags: Apply chilled eye gel ten minutes before making-up. Use make-up and techniques that draw attention to your upper eyelid: use plenty of mascara on the upper lashes only, and curl the upper lashes too.

Crêpey lines: Apply an eye cream containing cereal protein to tighten and therefore smooth the skin temporarily and to provide a good base. Use a matt rather than shimmery shadow on the lids, but try a little pale, shimmery shadow beneath the outer part of each brow so as to draw attention upwards, away from below the eyes.

MOUTH

Small: Put a lighter shade of lipstick all over your lips, then a darker one over the inner part of each lip.

Large: Put a darker shade of lipstick all over your lips, then a lighter one over the inner part of each lip.

SKIN

Uneven pigmentation: Either use a camouflage-type foundation all over, or disguise the pale patches with a concealer and then use an ordinary foundation all over.

Fine lines: Use a very light-textured, liquid foundation, or mix foundation with a little moisturizer before applying. Use either no powder or only a very light dusting of a translucent one.

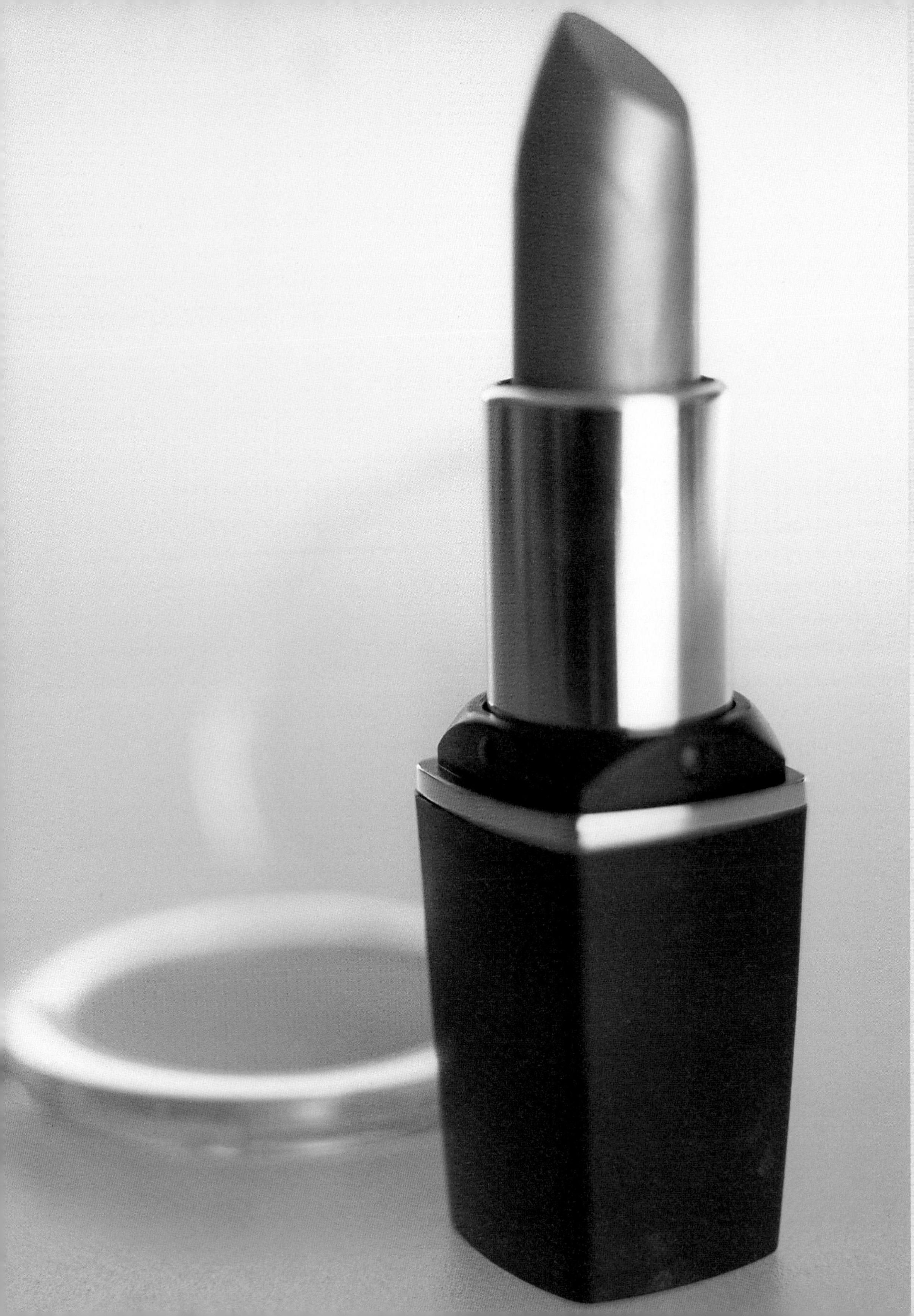

your gums and teeth

As soon as a person opens their mouth, it's apparent that the state of their gums and teeth can alter their whole appearance. For having healthy gums plus clean, shiny, straight teeth – with no large gaps or obvious fillings – gives the plainest of faces a wonderful lift.

Tooth decay and gum disease are the main enemies of good-looking, healthy teeth and gums. The main cause is the prolonged presence of acid around the teeth and gums. This comes from eating foods containing added sugar. Normal mouth bacteria consume traces of sugar remaining after swallowing the food. As they do this they release acids. These then start to dissolve the enamel that coats each tooth. The longer the acid remains, the more enamel is eroded. With repeated prolonged acid attack, the enamel may completely wear through in places, causing tooth decay.

The presence of plaque – a layer of food residue laden with bacteria, sugar and acid – around the gum margins makes gums inflamed unless removed within 24-36 hours. If this 'gingivitis' continues, the bone holding the teeth in place becomes inflamed; this 'periodontitis' eventually loosens teeth. Gum disease is most likely in people with thyroid disease or diabetes, in pregnant women, and in those with a dry mouth or on certain drugs. Researchers also believe that bacteria from diseased gums can enter the blood and raise the risk of premature birth, heart attacks and strokes.

KEEPING TEETH AND GUMS HEALTHY

This is how to keep teeth and gums healthy and looking good:

- Eat a healthy diet. This provides minerals such as calcium to rebuild enamel; beta-carotene, vitamins C and E, and zinc to combat inflammation; and fibre to clean teeth.
- Brush teeth twice daily to remove plaque. If brushing isn't practicable, either eat cheese or chew sugar-free gum to make your mouth water and so wash away food residues, or rinse your mouth well with plain water.
- Floss daily to remove food traces from between teeth.
- Avoid mouth-breathing, as this dries gums and raises the concentration of acid and sugar in saliva.
- Use effective stress-management to prevent a dry mouth and boost immunity, and exercise daily to boost immunity
- Look after your toothbrush: clean it well under running water each time you use it, and soak it sometimes in antiseptic solution. Bristles provide an ideal environment for bacteria, viruses and fungi to grow. Most of these micro-organisms are normally present in the mouth, but if you have a cold sore, or a gum or other mouth infection, or mouth ulcers, an unkempt brush will give these germs a place to multiply.
- Massage unhealthy gums each day with aloe vera gel; rinse with black tea or sage tea (made by pouring half a cup of boiling water over a teaspoon of dried sage); and take a daily dose of echinacea tincture.
- See your dentist regularly.

hair

The cut, condition and style of your hair make a surprisingly big difference to your face. Hair colour, too, alters how your facial skin and features look. And having attractive hair that boosts your image and personality can make your whole face appear brighter and more youthful.

One secret of discovering which hairstyle does most for you lies in discussion, experimentation and feedback from family, friends and professionals. Another lies in re-appraising every so often what you do with your hair, because its condition, growth rate, thickness and colour will alter from time to time throughout your life. This is because various situations affect the levels of nutrients and hormones that reach your scalp in the blood. Oestrogen, progesterone and testosterone affect the sebum-producing glands and hair roots in both men and women. And in women changes in their levels accompanying menstrual cycles, pregnancy and the menopause influence oiliness and thickness. Adequate levels of haemoglobin, the oxygen-carrying pigment in red blood cells, and thyroxine, from the thyroid gland, are essential for thick, healthy hair and the scalp's circulation affects its nourishment and oxygen supply.

Greying is caused by the loss of the natural pigmentation (with melanin) that occurs in the growing part of each hair's root. Your genes dictate to some extent when cells switch off their melanin-producing capacity. But other factors also play a part. Most important is a good blood supply to the hair roots so as to bring nutrients for pigmentation. Early greying can be attractive, but most people prefer to keep their natural colour as long as possible and to add colour to fading tones.

To help your hair give your face a natural lift:

- Get your cut, condition, style and colour sorted.
- Re-appraise these as often as necessary.
- Safeguard the scalp's blood supply by eating plenty of foods rich in essential fats, minerals (including silica), vitamin B, para-aminobenzoic acid (in mushrooms, spinach, wholegrain foods, molasses), oily fish and plant hormones (see Chapter 3).
- Avoid poor slimming diets, or too rapid a weight loss.
- Massage your scalp several times a week to boost its circulation and therefore bring more nutrients and oxygen.
- Stop smoking, as this makes arteries narrower, which reduces the blood supply to the scalp.
- Learn to manage stress effectively, as this helps maintain good circulation.
- Get some unfiltered daylight on your skin each day to optimize hormone production.
- Have thyroid hormone and haemoglobin tests if you notice your hair thinning, or have abnormal fatigue and weight gain.
- If you colour your hair as you grow older, choose a shade that's lighter than your previous natural hair colour, as this will be more flattering to your skin.
- Have fun with your hair sometimes – for example, by adding highlights, sparkles, plaits or ribbons.

clothes

What you wear has a big impact not just on your whole appearance, but also on the brightness of your skin, the shape of your face, the sparkle in your eye, and the colour of your hair. This is partly because of the colour of your clothes, partly because of their style, and partly because of your pleasure – or otherwise – in how you look.

COLOUR

Looking at skin with an artist's eye, you will see that its colour contains many tones. Some people have predominantly yellowish tones, in others pink predominates, and it is possible to see blue and green too. The balance of tones interacts visually with the colours you wear to give an effect that is more or less pleasing or flattering.

If you hold pieces of cloth of different colours below someone's face and ask several people to comment, there will be almost complete agreement on what looks best. Some colours obviously 'light up' an individual's face. Others seem to drain it of colour and brightness. These effects can be startlingly good or bad.

If you aren't sure what suits you best:

- Recall which outfits provoke compliments; these will probably be either because the colour lights up your skin or because the style is just right for your body shape.
- Ask a friend, or your mother or sister, to help you decide which colours are best.
- Visit a shop and hold various different-coloured garments in front of you in a mirror.
- Consult a colour adviser, such as one from Colour Me Beautiful (see page 157).
- Remember that something white or cream near the face can light it up. People with yellow skin tones often look better in cream, while those with bluish tones are usually favoured by white.

STYLE

Try different styles of trousers, skirts, jackets, shirts and jumpers from the ones you usually wear to see which do you most justice. Getting your clothes right can make a big difference not only to the way you look, but also to the way you feel about yourself. And feeling happy and self-confident naturally reflects in the expressions on your face.

ENJOYING YOUR CLOTHES

Dress for personal pleasure as well as for style and colour. Your clothes can be both an expression of your individuality and beautiful in their own right. And at best they will give you delight right through the day – as you choose your outfit and get dressed first thing, as you wear them about your daily business, and as you change for different activities. Conversely, as every one of us has probably experienced, there's nothing like knowing your clothes don't look good to cast a pall on the whole day.

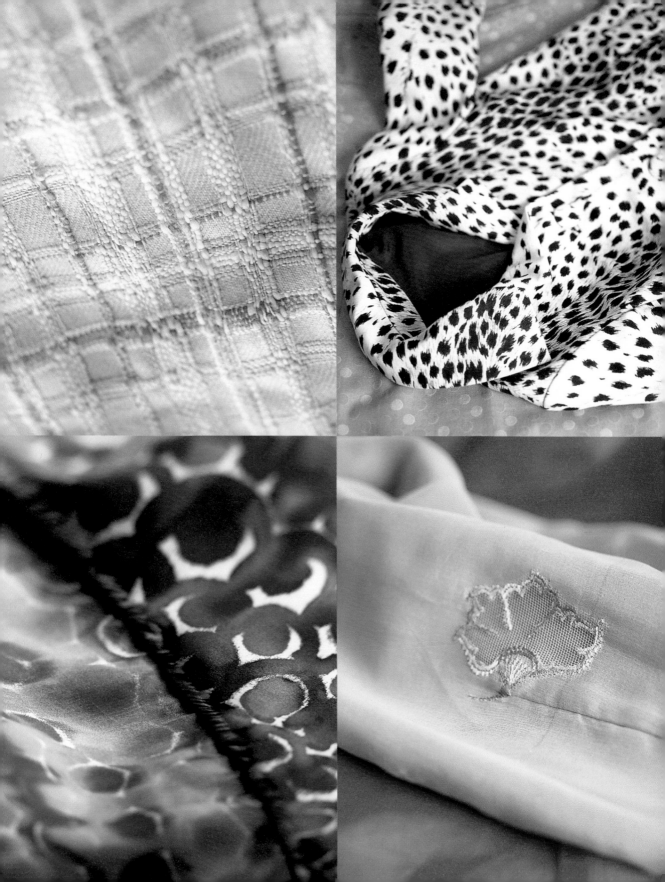

jewellery and other adornment

People in every culture throughout history have adorned their bodies in some way. Most of us enjoy developing the art and skills involved in painting our face, doing our hair and choosing our clothes. The practicalities involved in the routine of personal adornment become a familiar, welcome and relaxing part of our daily life. And choosing and wearing jewellery can add to our enjoyment.

Jewels themselves have, of course, always been symbolically important too. Precious stones such as emeralds, diamonds, sapphires and rubies represent wealth. And because of this – and because of the fact that they are beautiful in themselves – they are always highly prized. Historically men have bought jewels for their women – and still do – because they love them; they want to demonstrate their love in tangible terms and they also want to make their loved one look even lovelier. Some, of course, also want to display their weatlth and warn off the attention of other males. Rich women too buy precious jewellery, either because they like it and think it enhances their looks or because they want to show their material worth.

But of course you don't have to spend a fortune to enjoy jewellery. It's possible to buy attractively designed rings, bracelets, ear-rings, necklaces, watches and other pieces at a wide variety of costs, depending on what they are made from and the time that has gone into their design and manufacture.

CHOOSING JEWELLERY

When choosing jewellery, think in terms of two things: which colours and styles make you look good and which pieces you know you are going to enjoy. For when you love wearing a particular piece of jewellery, your very pleasure in knowing it is there will light up your face and give it a real lift.

Some people – often those with more obvious yellow tones in their skin – look their best when wearing gold. Others – generally those with blue tones – are more flattered by silver. If you are choosing a stone, go for the colour you like best, but before you decide, check it against your face. Depending on your skin tone, light turquoise ear-rings, for example, might look better than bright green ones on you. Or deep red ones may be preferable to pale pink.

Pearls near the face are always said to give a glow to the skin. But if you are choosing pearls, remember that they come in many different shades: pink, grey, creamy and even 'black'. And certain shades suit some people better than others.

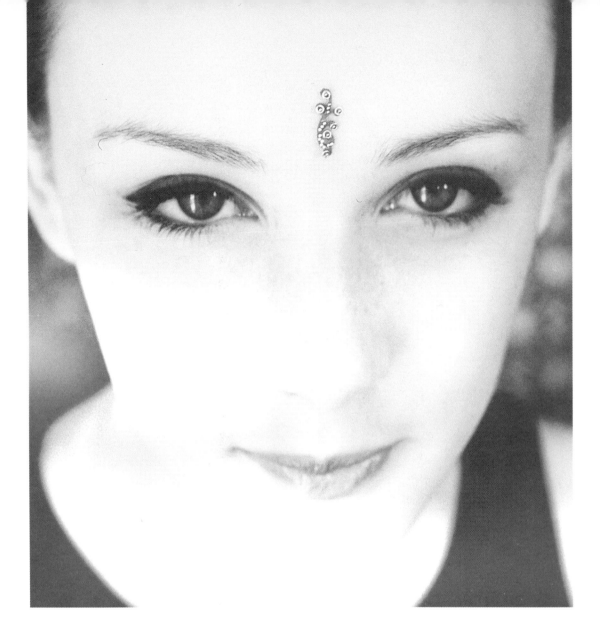

It can often be tempting to wear a piece of jewellery that is unflattering or unfashionable simply because it was expensive. Alternatively you might feel you should keep a certain item even when you don't like it, simply because someone special gave it to you. If this happens, consider having the piece remade by a jeweller to suit you better.

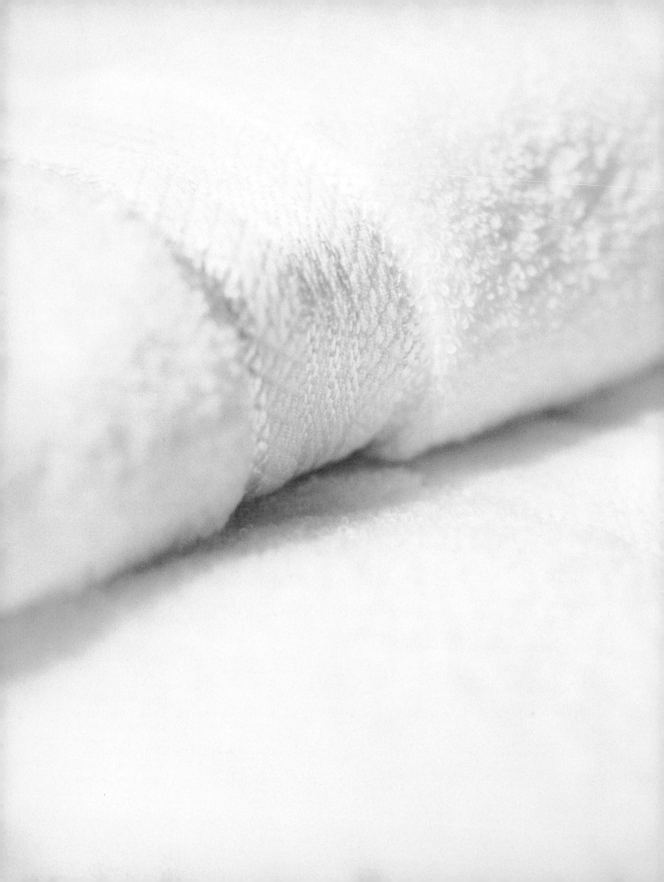

treating yourself
to a massage

The magic of massage is freely available any time. And a massage of the face – the part that most clearly reveals our personality and emotions – can bring a special sense of calmness and delight.

Massage is not only pleasurable but also an age-old way of comforting and healing. For comforting through touch comes naturally. We hold or hug our loved ones if they are upset. We rub a hurting place on ourselves until the pain eases. And we rest a hand on someone's shoulder if they are upset, to signify our support and concern.

Certain face-massage techniques have been passed down through the centuries because they are particularly soothing or useful for the face. And the good thing is that you can pick and choose one to use anywhere, any time, to help boost your circulation and lift away your stress.

the beauty of a face massage

A face massage can be wonderfully soothing, partly because stress so readily makes face muscles tense and partly, perhaps, because the experience reminds us of pleasurable times with our mother during infancy. So whether you do it yourself, or have someone do it for you, you'll probably end up feeling much more relaxed afterwards.

Healing someone through massage happens in several ways. First, by boosting the circulation of blood and lymph, massage brings more nutrients, oxygen and immune factors to the skin and speeds the removal of waste products like carbon dioxide. All this makes skin glow and reduces puffiness. Second, by giving pleasure, it increases the level of hormone-like substances called endorphins that make us feel and look better. Third, by relaxing tense muscles, it reduces the levels of stress hormones that result from muscle tension, immediately benefiting the circulation, blood pressure, heart rate, energy and joie de vivre. And fourth, by showing you care, it encourages emotional release and boosts self-esteem, lightening their step and making them feel loved and loveable In these ways massage works on mind, body and spirit.

QUICKIE FACE MASSAGES

Touch is a vital member of the five senses. The physical sensations experienced while being touched during a massage vary enormously. The pressure of the fingers may be firm, light or gentle. There may be continuous contact or repeated strokes, and the strokes may be feather-like or smooth and sweeping and – like music – rhythmical or unexpected, fast or slow, and growing softer or more pronounced.

We touch our own face many times every day, but receiving a face massage lets us experience touch in a different way. Whether we do it ourselves or enjoy the luxury of having it done, the gentle, intimate strokes can evoke memories of our mother's delight in us when we were babies, of a lover's timeless caress. The contrasting feelings of safety and vulnerability can combine with physical sensations and the energy flow between fingers and face to release deeply held emotions. And, more prosaically but no less important, a massage helps any excess tension in the face muscles to evaporate.

Reading about face massage may be inspiring, but having one is much more rewarding. So if the idea appeals or intrigues, why not plan a time soon for a full face massage, or do a 'quickie' face massage on yourself right now?

QUICKIE FACE MASSAGE 1 – THE ALL-OVER DESTRESSER

Relax yourself any time with this quickie 'All-over destresser' massage. All you need is some peace and quiet.

1 Sit comfortably on any chair, put your feet flat on the floor, legs uncrossed and your hands in your lap.

2 Take three long slow breaths, close your eyes and relax.

3 Cup your face with the heels of your hands cradling your chin.

4 Push your cupped hands gently upwards. Let your head sag so that your hands take a little of its weight. Be aware of the immediate sense of relaxation and comfort.

5 Move the flats of your hands slowly, lightly and gently, each making big sweeping circles over half your face. Lift them off almost completely in the downward half of each circle. Repeat ten times.

6 Tap lightly, with the middle three fingertips of each hand, from the chin and up the inner cheek to just below the eye. Do the same up the middle and outer parts of each cheek. Repeat three times.

7 Close your eyes, put these same three fingertips in a line across your forehead and press firmly for a while. Focus on the sensations in your forehead.

8 Finish by cupping your face as before.

QUICKIE FACE MASSAGE 2 – THE BUTTERFLY

Another quickie and an excellent stress-reliever, is the 'Butterfly'; this has the advantage of being easy to do any time.

1 Sit comfortably, legs uncrossed, feet flat on the floor and hands in your lap.

2 Take three long slow breaths and relax.

3 Stretch out your hands then, starting from your chin, use the flats of your fingertips to touch your skin very lightly and quickly, making repeated brushing movements (three or four a second) like the brushing of a butterfly wing. Move your fingers up your inner cheek each side to just below the eye. Then do the same up the middle and outer parts of each cheek.

4 Take the flats of your fingertips to the middle of your forehead, just above the bridge of your nose, and make the same movements up towards your hairline. Lift your fingertips and replace them, but this time a little out towards the side of the brow. Repeat the movements up towards your hairline, then with your fingertips starting above the outer part of the eyebrow each side.

5 Lastly, make similar movements all around each eye socket and over your closed eyes.

QUICKIE FACE MASSAGE 3 – THROUGH A COMPRESS

When you want a particularly relaxing and soothing quickie face massage, choose either the 'All-over destresser', or the 'Butterfly' massage, then prepare a moist compress. This can be warm or cool, and moistened with either herbal tea, or aromatherapy-oil-scented water.

1 Make a bowl of chamomile-flower herbal tea and cool to the required temperature. Or add two drops of neroli, rose or lavender oil to a bowl of water of the required temperature.

2 Soak a piece of cotton (of a suitable size to cover your face) in the bowl and gently wring the excess liquid from this compress.

3 Lie down comfortably and lay the moist compress over your face.

4 Now – over the compress – do steps 2–8 of the 'All-over destresser' massage, or steps 2–5 of the 'Butterfly' massage.

5 Remove the compress and put some moisturizer on your skin to seal in the remaining layer of moisture.

preparing for a full massage

A full face massage is even more relaxing and pleasurable than a quickie, and having someone do it for you is best of all. These guidelines are for the person giving the massage, but if you do it yourself, you can easily adapt them.

YOUR ENVIRONMENT

- Make the surroundings peaceful. Switch on the answer-phone and reduce its ringing-tone volume (or unplug the phone), and put a 'Do not disturb' sign on the door.
- Close the curtains and light candles if you like.
- Consider whether the air is too cold or too hot. The person you are massaging will need more warmth than you, because they will be relaxed and still.
- Choose some soothing music, preferably without words.
- Prepare a place for the person to lie. This could be a bed, sofa, massage-table or the floor. As the one doing the massage, you'll need room to sit with their head in front of you or, if using a massage-table, room to stand at its head.
- Cover the area with a large towel. Most massage-tables are narrow, which means the arms of the person being massaged readily slip off when they relax. Avoid this by placing a long towel across the table. When the person lies down, fold each end over an elbow, and tuck it well in under their body. This can make a surprisingly big difference to their comfort during the massage.
- Put another big towel nearby, ready to cover them and a blanket to add if they want to doze afterwards, because otherwise they may readily become uncomfortably chilled.
- Put a rolled-up towel ready to support their neck and have a box of tissues close by.

THE OIL

- Put two tablespoons of sweet-almond oil into a small, squeezable, plastic bottle, add four drops each of geranium and lavender oils and insert a stopper with a hole.
- Shake the bottle and stand it in a bowl of comfortably hot water to warm it up. It's never wise to use cold oil straight on the skin because it detracts from the feeling of comfort, trust and relaxation.

PREPARING YOURSELF AND YOUR SUBJECT

- You need loose clothes and a short-sleeved top; the person you are going to massage needs a loose-necked top.
- Remove rings, watch and bracelets and ask the person having the massage to take off any earrings, necklace, hair-band or glasses. They should also remove contact lenses if they use any.
- Check that your nails are smooth and your hands already warm. Cool hands are not pleasant on bare skin.
- Ask the person to lie on their back.
- Cover their body with a towel for warmth even though they are clothed.
- Ask if they would like some music.
- Sit comfortably, with their head in front of you. Relax by taking some slow deep breaths, then focus on the waiting person.

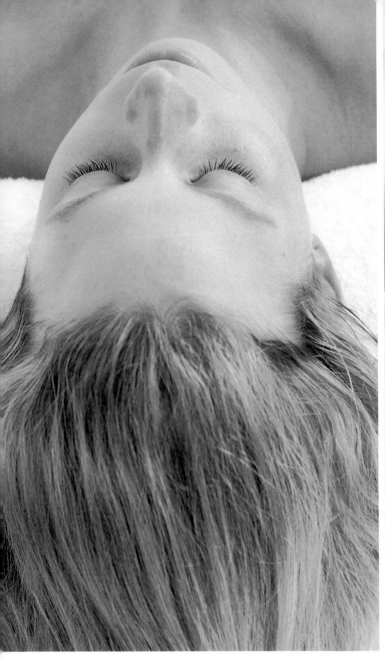

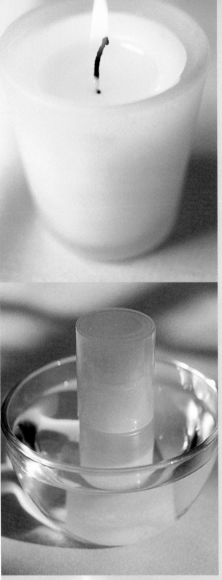

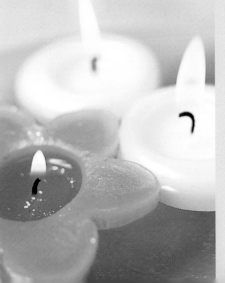

ABOVE

Prepare a place for the person to lie. This might be a bed, sofa, massage table, or the floor. As masseur, you will need room to sit with their head in front of you and, if using a massage-table, room to stand at its head end. A rolled-up towel should be used to support the head.

TOP RIGHT AND BOTTOM

Create a calm and peaceful environment. Unplug the phone and choose some soothing music. Draw the curtains and use some candles for soft lighting.

MIDDLE

Use a blend of sweet almond, geranium and lavender oils for the full face massage. Stand the oil in a bowl of comfortably hot water to ensure that it is not too cold on the skin.

103

know your essential oils

Certain essential plant oils are particularly appropriate for using (see pages 108–9) on your face. This may be because of their effects on your skin, your mind, your body, or all three.

Add eight drops of your chosen oil to two tablespoons of base oil (see page 113). To some extent almost every essential oil boosts cell-regeneration, has antiseptic properties, and stimulates the local circulation.

Chamomile (Roman): This oil soothes irritated, inflamed skin and calms itching. It's a good choice for sensitive or inflamed skin, and for those with tense facial muscles. It goes well with geranium and lavender, but as its fragrance notes are predominantly 'middle, some of the best choices for blends are cedarwood, clary sage, frankincense, jasmine, neroli, rose and ylang ylang.

Clary Sage: Though its scent is certainly not to everyone's taste, many people report that clary sage encourages relaxation and helps lift depression, especially if this is associated with anxiety and stress. It's reputed to be a good 'women's' oil, as it contains oestrogen-like substances called diterpenes that may exert a beneficial effect on the skin. The fragrance has a top-to-middle note which blends well with the base notes of cedarwood, frankincense, jasmine, neroli, rose, ylang ylang and sandalwood.

Frankincense: An oil that is said to aid cell regeneration and counter premature ageing, and scarring. It is also said to inspire a relaxed and meditative mood, which is why it's used to make the incense that is burnt in some churches. However, while some love it, others really don't like its rich heavy smell one bit. Its fragrance blends well with neroli and sandalwood, but its base note means it also goes well with chamomile, clary sage, geranium, juniper berry and lavender.

Geranium: You either love or hate this smell. If you like it, its female-friendly properties may be especially helpful when hormone levels are changing rapidly, such as before periods or around the menopause, possibly due to the effect of oestrogen-like substances (diterpenes) on the skin. Its aroma relaxes or stimulates, according to your need, and helps lift depression. The fragrance goes well with juniper berry, but has a middle note, so also blends well with cedarwood, clary sage, frankincense, jasmine, neroli, rose, sandalwood and ylang ylang.

Jasmine: This intensely sweet oil is expensive, much favoured by perfumers, and renowned for being mentally uplifting. It's also said to have aphrodisiac properties and to be useful in skin products for ageing skin. Jasmine complements most oils - especially neroli, rose and sandalwood - very well, but the base note of its fraagrance means it blends especially well with cardamom, chamomile, clary sage, geranium, juniper berry and lavender.

Lavender: This delightful oil conjures the warmth of summer sun and the scent of freshly laundered linen. It encourages skin-cell regeneration, so it can benefit ageing or damaged skin; it can also help relax mental and physical tension and lighten depression. Lavender partners most oils well, but its fragrance has a middle note, so it's particularly good with cedarwood, clary sage, frankincense, jasmine, neroli, rose, sandalwood and ylang ylang.

Neroli: The pleasure derived from the light, sweet, heavenly scent of this citrus oil - extracted from the blossoms of the bitter orange tree - is just one of the reasons why it is so good for relieving stress and stress-related conditions, including some depression and sleep problems. It's also a good choice for encouraging cell regeneration in ageing skin. Neroli is lovely with all oils, but as its fragrance note is base, it's a good partner for chamomile, clary sage, geranium, juniper berry and lavender

FOR OILY SKIN

These oils are the ones to choose if your skin is oily:

Cardamom: A sweet-spicy oil that has a stimulating action on the local circulation; this may help make the skin brighter and clearer. It is reputed to have anti-fatigue and aphrodisiac qualities.

Cedarwood: Another oil that is said to stimulate the skin even while at the same time its woody-balsamic fragrance promotes sleep.

Cypress: Another relaxing oil that is traditionally used for greasy skin and for acne. Its lovely 'smokey' and balsamic smell also promotes sleep.

Rose: Although expensive, the anti-ageing properties of rose oil make it an excellent aid for keeping skin fresh, dewy and youthful. It is also one of the best-loved oils and is celebrated as an aphrodisiac. Use one drop in home-made massage oils or other skin products. Rose goes particularly well with jasmine, neroli and sandalwood. But the base note of its fragrance also makes it a good partner for chamomile, clary sage, geranium, juniper berry and lavender.

Ylang ylang: The sweet fragrance of ylang ylang makes it useful for lifting the sadness and yearning that can distort the face in times of mourning. It is traditionally recommended for dry and sensitive skin. Ylang ylang is a good partner for jasmine, rose and sandalwood, but as its fragrance has a base note, it also goes well with chamomile, clary sage, geranium, juniper berry and lavender.

Juniper berry: A stimulating oil that is also good if you are feeling depressed.

Sandalwood: This gentle oil is a good choice not only for those with particularly greasy skin, and with acne, but also for those with other skin types, including ageing skin, and skin subject to a high colour, including rosacea (see page 138). Inhaling its woody-balsamic fragrance can promote relaxation.

Caution: dilute all essential oils – other than frankincense or lavender – with a base oil (see page 113) before use.

giving a full face massage

Before you begin, remind yourself that the individual you are about to massage trusts you to touch them gently and with respect. And because the intimacy involved in receiving a face massage sometimes brings up deep emotions, be prepared for them to want to talk, laugh or even cry.

1 Put two to three drops of warmed oil into the palm of one hand, place the bottle within easy reach, but where you won't knock it over, and rub your palms lightly together. *Enhance the soothing nature of the massage by maintaining physical contact with the person you are massaging all the time. If you need more oil, lightly rest one hand, palm-up, on the person's cheek. With the other squeeze some oil from the bottle on to your waiting palm, then, still resting on the cheek, rub your palms together.*

Topping up the amount of oil on your hands this way means the person you are massaging never feels ignored or, more perturbingly, abandoned.

2 Cup your subject's face with your fingertips meeting beneath the chin. Rest a while and mark the beginning by softly saying something like, 'Hello, Mary, this is for you.' *Hearing your name spoken at this early stage of the massage can make the experience even more personal and may bring up memories, at a deep level, of early childhood.*

Let the person decide whether to talk. Some like talking; others prefer silence. Sometimes a massage feels so deeply intimate that it can trigger emotions. The person may cry, or disclose memories, concerns or challenges. A few people for whom this is their first face massage feel giggly, jumpy or awkward until they relax and start to enjoy the experience.

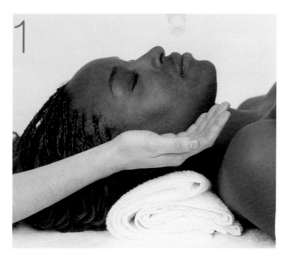

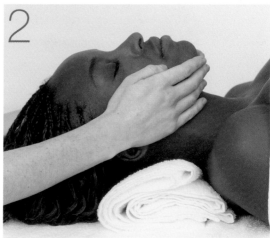

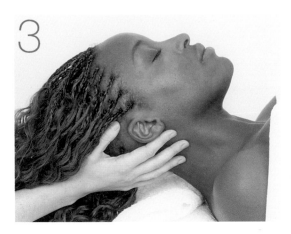

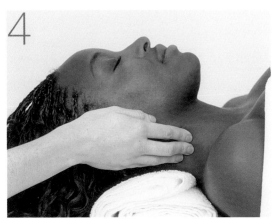

3 Slide your hands slowly down the sides of the neck, then cup the head from underneath. Lift it up, pull it towards you a little and gently set it down again. This helps the neck and shoulder muscles relax. Repeat twice. *The head weighs 4.5–6 kg (10–13 lbs). Not surprisingly, many people, especially those with desk jobs who lean over their work, have a lot of tension in the neck and shoulders. This encourages facial tension.*

4 Massage the muscles between the neck and shoulders. Start by stroking, then knead them firmly. Work up the sides of the neck, gently stroking the long bands of muscle here several times, then work on them with small, firm, circular movements. *By now the person should be feeling pleasantly cosseted. Replenish the oil if necessary, then cup the face again as in step1.*

5 Using the middle three fingertips of each hand, work around the jaw from the chin to the jaw joint just in front of the ear, using small, light but firm, circular movements. Repeat.

The jaw muscles are particularly prone to tension. Triggers include stress, draughts, hugging the phone in the crook of your neck, a poor dental 'bite', a heavy shoulder bag and grinding the teeth without realising while asleep at night.

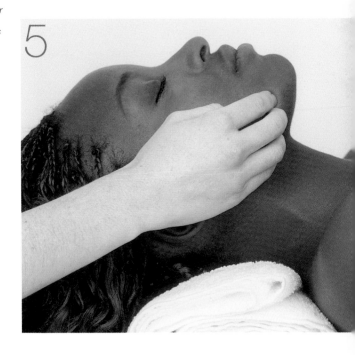

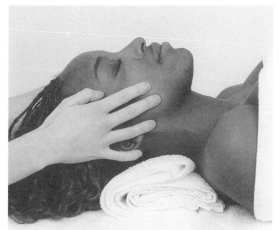

6 Use very small, light but firm strokes of the middle three fingers of each hand to make a series of lines, each starting on the chin and fanning up and out over the cheeks. Gradually cover the whole area, never dragging the skin. *This eases tension and stimulates the circulation. Remember to stay relaxed yourself.*

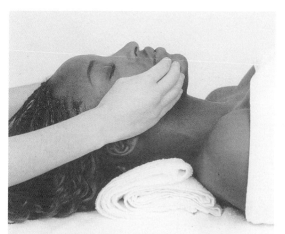

7 Place the middle three fingertips of each hand above the upper lip and massage with tiny firm circular movements towards the corners of the mouth. Continue under the mouth towards the midline. *You may notice their mouth opening slightly. This shows they're feeling relaxed.*

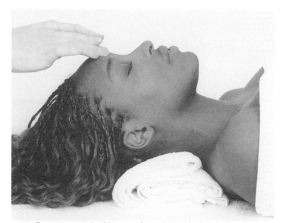

8 Put the middle fingers of each hand above the corners of the mouth, then trace slowly and lightly up the sides of the nose, on to the bridge and up to the forehead. Quickly return them to the starting position. Repeat six or seven times. *This links the massage of the lower and upper part of the face.*

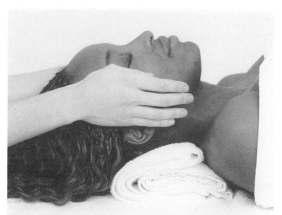

9 Put the heels of your hands lightly but firmly on the middle of the forehead, touching each other. Keep your fingers lifted off the face. Slowly slide your hands away from each other, following the contours of the forehead and ironing out any skin creases, until they reach the hairline. Repeat several times. *This stretches out any vertical frown lines.*

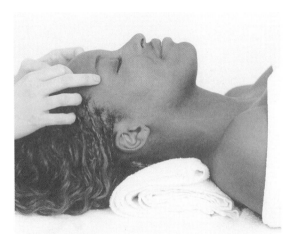

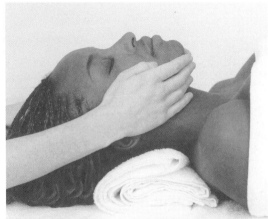

10 With both your middle fingertips, make light firm circles around the eyes: start at the bridge of the nose, continue across the browbones and then extremely lightly, over the upper cheekbones and back to the nose. Repeat several times. Lastly, cover the eyes lightly with your palms for half a minute or so. *This encourages a deep feeling of relaxation.*

11 End the massage by cupping the person's face again for a while, as in step 1, and saying something softly and meaningfully to end the session, such as 'Mary, you're a very special person.' or 'May your day ahead be all you want it to be.' *Hearing such words spoken after the intimacy of a face massage can have a surprising significance, so choose carefully and in your knowledge of the person.*

AFTER THE MASSAGE

When you've finished the massage, lay an extra blanket or a thick towel over the person's body. This is because their whole body will probably be extremely relaxed. This may make them feel sleepy and it is possible that they will actually fall into a very deep sleep for a short while, if they are allowed. Unless you provide some extra covering their metabolic rate may decrease enough to make them feel chilly, however warm they were at first and however warm the room.

Softly say they are welcome (assuming this is indeed the case) to have a sleep if they wish and then, if necessary, add some idea of how long this sleep can be. Quietly put the lids on the oil bottles and leave the room if possible. When you return, enter calmly, put a hand on their shoulder and speak gently if you need to wake them, then help them return to normal life without too big a jolt by talking about ordinary everyday things, or, perhaps, their experience of the massage.

Some people like to 'swap' face massages, by first one giving the other a massage, then when they have finished, the other giving them one. This is fine, but does mean that the option of a sleep is curtailed, at least for the first to be massaged.

complementary therapies

The skin can benefit from many of the natural things around us, of which four – plants, water, light and sound – are particularly important. Plant roots, stems, leaves, flowers and seeds provide us with oils and other healing extracts for aromatherapy, and for herbal and flower remedies. Water – just as it is, cold, warm or hot, or in steam or compresses – enables us to perform hydrotherapy. Light, or one or more of its component wavelengths, gives us bright-light, ultra-violet and colour therapies. Even sound waves can have surprisingly beneficial effects.

In this chapter we'll see how these natural therapies can help prevent premature ageing of the skin and boost its natural radiance and resilience. We'll look at how you can use them at home, on yourself or on your friends and family. And we'll also consider both osteopathy and the use of electricity.

aromatherapy

Aromatherapy uses plant oils as they are, or to enrich creams and other skin-care products. These so-called 'essential' oils contain the healing essence of a plant and can be added to massage oil to aid relaxation and boost circulation. Essential oils extracted from plants contain a combination of naturally occurring chemicals; the range and combination of these accounts for each oil's unique fragrance and healing qualities.

Aromatherapy works in three ways.

The first is by the inhalation and absorption through the lungs of the oil's vapour. When you inhale, aromatic molecules drift to the top of your nose, where they stimulate nerve endings that report to the brain. If the smell reminds you of a previous time when you smelt something similar, and if that was pleasing, relaxing or stimulating, you will probably experience the same benefits again. Some of these molecules act on very 'primitive' parts of the brain to produce profound effects. At the same time aromatic molecules from the oil can pass through the lining of the nose and breathing passages into your blood. Here they circulate to the rest of the body where they can influence the behaviour of, for example, the immune system, the hormone-producing glands, and the brain and nerves.

The second mechanism behind aromatherapy is the absorption through the skin of small oil molecules. These act both within the skin and, more generally, by passing through the skin into the blood. Tests can register them in the blood within minutes of applying aromatherapy oil. However, you absorb more of an essential oil's active ingredients by inhaling its aroma than you do by smoothing it on your skin, which proves the aptness of the term 'aromatherapy'.

The third way in which aromatherapy works is by the action of the hands. The smoothing or massaging in of an oil can be slow and gentle, to soothe and relax, or faster and firmer, to stimulate and warm. And in addition to the physical benefits of this skin-to-skin contact, the emotional intimacy involved in having someone else massage you can in itself be surprisingly beneficial.

Because of aromatherapy's de-stressing effects, and the fact that some of an essential oil's potent molecules enter the skin and pass into the blood, many of these oils benefit the face either when used directly on it, or when applied elsewhere.

Buy essential oils from pharmacies, health shops and many supermarkets, or by mail-order (see page 156). A good guide is to choose the ones whose smell you like.

The following oils are especially good to use – usually diluted – for your face or body:

Lavender	Neroli	Clary sage
Ylang ylang	Rose	Chamomile
Geranium	Jasmine	Frankincense

Useful ones for oily skin include:

| Cardamom | Sandalwood | Cedarwood |
| Cypress | Juniper berry | |

For descriptions of all of these oils, see pages 104–5. You also need some 'base' oil for diluting essential oils if they are not already diluted by the supplier. These are some of the ones most commonly used:

Sweet-almond   Jojoba   Grapeseed

Macadamia nut   Peach-kernel   Apricot-kernel

Wheatgerm

For descriptions of all of these oils, see pages 104–5.

There are various ways of using essential oils. Try adding them to a home-made skin product (see the recipes on pages 30–41) or stirring a few drops into a commercial product. The amount you use depends on the product's volume and nature. For example, stir one to two drops of undiluted oil into a full 100-ml (3$\frac{1}{2}$-fl-oz) pot; if this is not fragrant enough, add another few drops.

Prepare oil for a facial massage by adding eight drops of neat essential oil to two tablespoons of base oil. When it comes to your bath, make it smell lovely by adding five to ten drops of essential oil to a full bath. Alternatively, encourage the oil to disperse better by adding a mixture of either five to ten drops of essential oil blended into a teaspoon of base oil, or five to ten drops of essential oil blended into a teaspoon of moisturizer.

Pages 40–41 explain how to incorporate essential oils into home-made 'anti-wrinkle' patches or compresses.

Benefit from the scent of essential oils in a room by using a ceramic oil burner. Add up to five drops of essential oil to the water in the container, then light the night-light candle below.

If pregnant, use only lavender, citrus (neroli, bergamot, grapefruit, petitgrain, orange, lime), frankincense or ylang ylang oils. There is a very slight though unproven suspicion that other oils might provoke miscarriage or damage the baby, but the oils specified are considered perfectly safe. If using citrus oil, keep sunlight off oiled skin for twenty-four hours, as otherwise certain substances called psoralens in the oil could provoke a light-sensitive rash. Dilute all essential oils other than tea tree, frankincense and lavender before using on the skin.

When buying aromatherapy oils, be aware of exactly what you are buying. Many oils are sold pre-diluted in a base oil. This has both pros and cons. The good thing is that you may be able to use the oil directly on your skin or in your bath, for example, without diluting it in a base oil yourself first. However, the actual dilution is usually not stated, so the oil may be very much more dilute than you would wish, and the base oil may be a very cheap one and not the one you would ideally choose. Ideally it's best to buy essential oils and base oils separately and from a reputable supplier. Store all your oils in a dark, cool place to help keep them in good condition.

herbal and flower remedies

Plants contain many substances useful for enhancing, soothing and healing skin, quite apart from the essential oils already described. Such substances include vitamins, minerals, essential fats and a wide variety of potent antioxidants – including brightly coloured pigments such as flavonoids in fruits and vegetables (with citrus flavonoids some of the most potent), proanthocyanidins (in blueberries, elderberries and blackberries) and resveratrol and polyphenols (in black grapes).

Some plants, such as aloe vera, contain active ingredients that help skin retain moisture and aid the healing of sunburned or other inflamed skin. Others, such as comfrey and aloe vera again, contain substances that encourage new skin and connective tissue cells to grow. And there is a lot of interest in beauty circles in alpha-hydroxy acids – fruit are present in a wide variety of fruits and used for exfoliating and smoothing skin.

For some cosmetic or healing purposes you use the whole plant or its parts, fresh or dried. You might, for example, eat them as a food, add them to bath water or put them in a poultice. For others you use a tea, an extract or an alcoholic tincture made from the roots, stems, leaves, flowers, seeds, bark or all the aerial (above-ground) parts.

Consider growing herbs such as lemon balm, mint and aloe vera in your garden, in a tub or window box, or on a window sill. Alternatively, buy fresh or dried herbs, or ready-made remedies, from a supermarket, pharmacy, plant nursery or health store.

The best time for harvesting leaves, flowers or other plant parts is the first thing in the morning, because this is the time of day when the plant's sap rises, and when many of the substances in the plant that act on the skin are therefore at their highest levels. Reputable herbal companies are well aware of the need to sell herbs with high levels of active ingredients, and if you visit a herb farm at harvest time you'll probably be struck by the high level of attention to detail that accompanies every part of the process.

If you want to use fresh herbs to make a herbal tea or oil, for example, pick the leaves or harvest the other plant parts you need as near the time of making the product as possible. And always handle them very gently. These precautions help ensure that the levels of active ingredients remain high. If you intend drying or otherwise preserving fresh herbs, don't leave them lying around after being picked, but spread them out so they can dry naturally, then package them up straight away so they retain as much strength as possible.

Use up herbal tea within a few hours of making it, if possible, and meanwhile store it in the fridge. As for dried herbs, herbal oils and flower essences, whether they are home-produced or bought from a shop, it is best to store them in a dark, cool, dry place where their active ingredients will be preserved for as long as possible.

Always check the use-by date on any herbal product you have bought, and buy anew if necessary.

Herbal teas and oils, as well as flower essences, make good beauty aids and you can easily make teas and oils yourself at home.

HERBAL TEAS

To make a tea suitable for moistening a compress (see pages 40–41), using as a neck splash (see page 148) , adding to your bathwater or drinking (to care for the skin from within), use a herbal teabag as directed on the packet, or use fresh or dried herbs as follows:

Put 55g (2oz) fresh or 25g (1oz) dried plant parts in a pot or bowl. Fill with 600ml (1 pint/2¼ cups) boiling water, cover, steep for ten minutes, then strain and use.

To make tea from bark, seeds or roots such as carrots, first chop or crush the material:

Put 55g (2oz) fresh or 25g (1oz) dried plant parts in a saucepan, add a little over 600ml (1 pint/2½ cups) of water, simmer for fifteen minutes and strain.

HERBAL OIL

To make a healing herbal oil – from, for example, bright yellow St John's wort (hypericum) flowers – you need to dissolve the plant's goodness in the oil, so combine the herbs with oil as follows:

Put a handful of the herb into a screw-top jar, such as a 450-g (1-lb) jam jar, fill with sweet-almond oil and screw on the lid. Leave on a window sill (sunny if possible) and shake every day for two weeks. Strain through muslin and squeeze out the rest of the oil from the herb (now in the cloth). Put the oil into a dark bottle and store in a cool, dark cupboard.

FLOWER ESSENCES

As for flowers, simply seeing, feeling or smelling them can soothe away stress. A flower's healing power can also be harnessed by extracting its essential oil or preparing an alcoholic extract (tincture) called a flower essence.

The first range of flower essences to be marketed were the Bach (pronounced 'Batch') remedies in the UK, though now many countries have their own ranges, made from flowers indigenous to each country. Dr Edward Bach was interested in people's moods and feelings and used intuition and observation to develop thirty-seven floral extracts. You choose one or more according to how you are feeling emotionally. One important way they work is through you having to recognize your emotions as you choose what to take.

For example, for:

- depression from sad or negative thoughts: choose honeysuckle or star of Bethlehem
- general depression: choose mustard or wild rose
- fear: choose aspen
- jealousy or anger: choose holly
- under-confidence: choose larch
- tiredness or stress: choose olive.

To use the flower essence, put two drops of the essence you have chosen into a glass of water and sip during the day. Alternatively, put two drops of each of up to seven essences in a 27-ml (1-fl oz) dropper bottle, add a teaspoon of brandy or glycerine, fill up with spring water and take four drops of this four times a day.

acupressure

Acupressure boosts the circulation of blood, tissue fluid and lymph, making your face look clearer and brighter and, perhaps, helping to prevent premature ageing. It can also relieve muscle tension, so its regular use may help to prevent premature lines.

Facial acupressure involves pressing certain points on the face with the tip of the thumb or finger. This is said to encourage a type of energy, qi or chi (pronounced 'chee'), to flow freely along hypothetical 'channels' in the body called meridians. There are said to be twelve major meridians, each named after a particular organ, plus two others. The energy flow can be normal, blocked, overactive or weak. Stimulation of acupressure points (acupoints) is believed to encourage a normal flow.

Several findings support this. Many acupoints are over tiny bony depressions where a nerve or blood vessel passes close to the skin and there is a lower electrical resistance here than in the surrounding skin. Also, many acupoints correspond with the tender, tense, hard bands or knots (myofascial trigger points) that some people get in their muscles, fascia (fibrous sheets of tissue) or tendons. Massaging these relieves both local tenderness and radiating pain.

Here are three types of acupressure to try:

- Press to increase (tonify) the energy flow: press with thumbtip or fingertip for two minutes, imagining the acupoint as a funnel filling with energy.
- Pump with thumbtip or fingertip for two minutes, or rotate in little circles, to release a blocked energy flow and, perhaps, relieve local muscle tension.
- Stroke with featherlight fingertips to calm an excessive energy flow.

Whether you treat yourself to regular – perhaps weekly – acupressure, or have someone else do it for you, breathe freely and relax as much as possible. If treating yourself, stop every so often to check that you are not over-tensing your arm. Increase the benefit by smoothing in some moisturizing cream (see pages 36–7) or facial massage oil (see page 104) first.

Use the picture opposite to locate each point. And remember that you may feel a small depression or notice a slight tingle as you press. Start by pressing point 1 for five seconds, then pumping or rotating twenty times; alternatively, if you feel stressed but your muscles are not tense, stroke it. Repeat on each point around your eyes, cheeks, mouth, chin and jaw. When there is a symmetrical pair of points, press them with your left and right fingers at the same time. Work on any tender points for longer; tenderness may indicate a disrupted energy flow, and acupressure can relieve the discomfort.

RIGHT
The spots on this woman's face represent the points that are traditionally used as acupressure points. Many of them come in symmetrical pairs, one of each pair on either side of the face, and many of them correspond with tiny notches in the skin that you can locate with the tip of your finger.

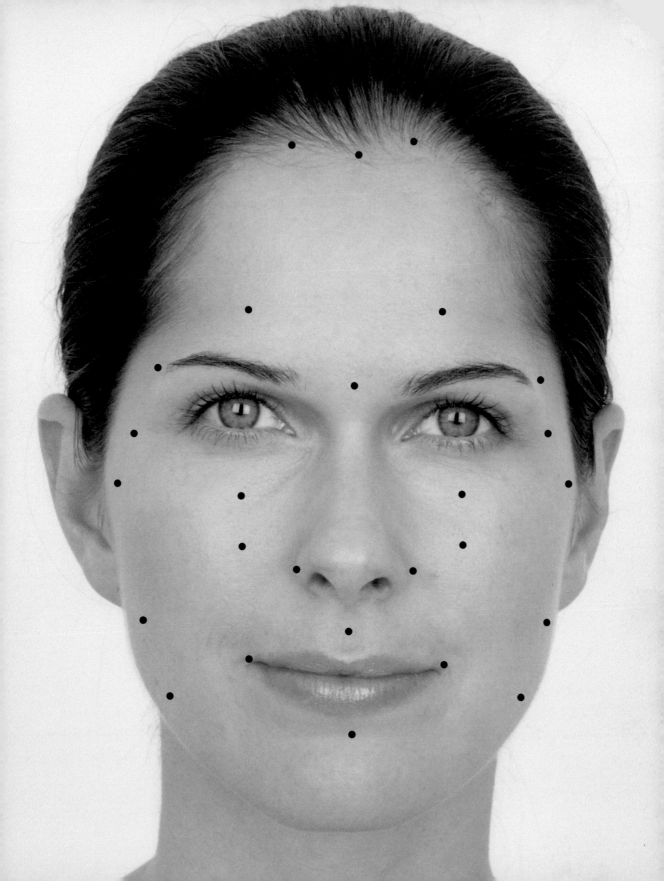

heat and cold water therapy

People have boosted health and well-being with heat, cold and water for millennia. Water can have powerful healing effects. And even just looking at natural forms of water – such as streams, waterfalls, icicles, snow-covered mountains, mists and rainbows – can induce a sense of awe and wonder and, at the very least, make us relax.

The combination of heat or cold, and water, as in a bath or shower, sea or pool, jacuzzi, sauna, steam room or hot tub, can benefit us physically and emotionally and have positive effects on our face by boosting our circulation and immunity. We can also treat our face to a facial sauna, compress, or herbal or floral splash. And you can release the skin-friendly properties of oatmeal, essential oils and other herbal extracts by dissolving, suspending or floating them in water.

Heat tends to relax tense facial muscles and may soothe inflamed skin, while something cool makes a hot, sweaty face more comfortable, stimulates a sluggish circulation and helps prevent puffy eyes. Some facial pains respond to heat, others to cold, with several problems being particularly responsive to a change in temperature.

Here are some ways of applying water to your face.

DIRECT HEAT ON FACE

Tense face muscles such as those around an aching jaw joint may relax with the heat from a safely covered hot-water bottle, an electric heating pad, or a microwaved hot pack.

DIRECT COLD ON FACE

A headache that has spread to your forehead or temples may ease with the application of an ice pack. Try using some ice cubes in a plastic bag (secured so that it cannot leak and wrapped in a towel so that it will not burn your skin). Alternatively, and more simply, use a packet of frozen peas.

FACIAL COMPRESS

A sore, dry or lined area of your face may well respond to treatment with an appropriate herbal or aromathearpy compress (see pages 40–41).

FACIAL SPLASH

Ageing skin will benefit from a gentle splash with room-temperature rose water (see page 33) in the morning. Wait until nearly dry, then apply some moisturizer to seal in a fine layer of scented droplets.

FACIAL 'SAUNA'

A dry, prematurely lined or pimply face may benefit from a facial 'sauna', also known as a facial steam bath. Fill a 600-ml (1-pint/2½-cup) bowl three-quarters full with boiling water. For dry or prematurely lined skin, add four drops of rose or geranium essential oil to the water. For pimply skin, add five drops of tea tree oil. Lean over the bowl with a towel over both your head and the bowl, and let the scented steam bathe your face for ten minutes. Seal a layer of regenerating healing mist to your skin afterwards by smoothing a little moisturizer in.

COLD WATER THERAPY

A cold facial splash can certainly be very refreshing at the time. But many people believe that the regular immersion of their whole body in cold water makes them feel better in the long term too. As we've seen, anything that makes you feel good reduces your stress level and boosts the blood-levels of natural 'feel-good' substances such as endorphins.

This feel-good effect is one reason why so many Europeans flock to spas for cold water therapy; why Scandinavians and, increasingly, others too, enjoy a cold shower after each session in the sauna; and why some people sea-bathe all year round.

The other reason is they believe – or their doctors or other therapists tell them – that immersion in cold water can help a variety of health problems. The possible benefits of cold-water therapy have been discussed since Roman times, but the interesting thing is there is now increasing medical evidence to back this up this belief that it has positive effects. Researchers have increasing evidence that regular immersion in cold water affects not just a person's sense of well-being, but also their health and energy. And some of their findings are surprising.

A daily cold-water bath alters the body's circulation and chemistry for several hours. It boosts the circulation to the liver, gut, kidneys, ovaries and other organs, and raises the levels of many hormones, including oestrogen, progesterone, and thyroxine. It also stimulates several immune-system cells, and may help prevent potentially dangerous blood clots in arteries and veins. This is all valuable to the whole body, including the skin of the face, its blood vessels, nerves and other structures, and its underlying muscles.

Researchers are continuing their studies to assess whether such changes can, among other things:

- Increase resistance to infection.
- Burn off body fat.
- Lower the level of low-density lipoprotein cholesterol (the type that can be bad news if chemically altered (oxidized) by such things as a poor diet, inflammation or stress).
- Aid fertility problems by increasing sex hormone levels.
- Lessen depression.
- Help those with the chronic fatigue syndrome (formerly known as myalgic encephalomyelitis, or ME). This is associated with more than six months of aching muscles, and episodes of unwarranted and sometimes disabling exhaustion. There may be headaches; poor sleep, concentration, memory and temperature control; and a one in two risk of depression; and irritable bowel syndrome is three times as likely).

If you wish to try cold water therapy, have your cold bath in the morning, make sure the room is warm, and always take care to get into the bath slowly so as not to get a shock. This is how to do it:

1 Start by adjusting the water temperature to 20°C, and stay in it, submerged up to your chin, for five minutes.

2 Gradually, over a period of 12 weeks, decrease the temperature by a degree at a time, to 16°C, and increase the time you stay in the water to 20 minutes.

If you feel better with a daily cold bath, continue doing it after this three-month trial.

Caution: see your doctor first if you have heart disease, high blood pressure, or other long-term illness.

light therapy

Visible light includes red, orange, yellow, green, blue, indigo and violet wavelengths, whereas the ultra-violet rays of light are often largely invisible. Light can have powerfully beneficial effects on you and your skin (but see also pages 24–5).

Good health depends on our body being exposed to a certain amount of bright white light. This makes our eyes send messages to the hypothalamus and pineal gland in the brain, which in turn influence many hormones, affecting sleep, menstrual periods, fertility, the body clock and our mental well-being. Light may also lower a high blood

cholesterol level. This helps the skin if its arteries are becoming clogged up with a fatty layer of oxidized low-density-lipoprotein cholesterol (atheroma). This is because less blood flows through narrowed arteries, so less oxygen and nutrients get to the skin.

Ultra-violet (UV) rays promote vitamin-D production in the skin,

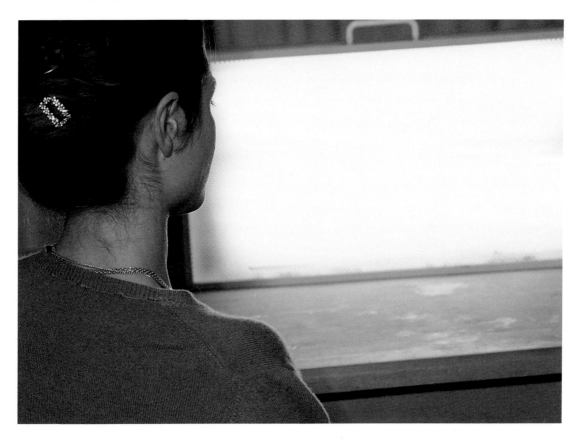

boost production of natural 'feel-good' substances called endorphins, and kill skin bacteria. Light aids the absorption of active ingredients in skin-care products by the skin. And light is itself absorbed by the skin as photons – packets of energy that provoke electro-chemical changes in the skin.

Coloured wavelengths are like nutrients: we need each one of them for good health. Their energy influences different cells in different ways. 'Full-spectrum' white light has 'full' helpings of colours, and comes from the sun in clear weather at midday. But white light from morning or evening sunlight, and most electric light, lacks certain colours. So spend at least fifteen minutes outdoors (taking care not to burn) each day; in winter, when the sun is at its weakest, do this around midday.

Certain skin problems benefit from using – or avoiding – particular colours. Try using a 'warm' (reddish) lightbulb or tube for depression, fatigue or poor circulation; or a 'cool' (bluish) one for stress, high blood pressure or inflammation.

Experiment further with by using bright-coloured light on your face or body. Put a coloured transparent gel (acetate sheet) from an art supply shop over a spotlight (with a gap to prevent over-heating). Use a blue gel to soothe stress and infection; red to increase collagen and elastin in sagging skin, bring more blood to cold areas, aid healing or treat inflammation; yellow for fatigue; and green to encourage the drainage of tissue fluid and lymph in puffy places. Sit 0.6–1.2m (2-4ft) away, for fifteen minutes for a blue gel, seven for a red, twelve for a yellow, and fifteen for a green. Balance this with a shorter time in front of a 'complementary' colour: after a blue gel, use a red one for three minutes; after a red, a blue for three; after a yellow, a violet for six; and after a green, a magenta for seven.

(Avoid red light if you have high blood pressure.)

Alternatively, use a coloured beam made by sticking a small piece of coloured gel over a bright pen-torch bulb. Focus it on acupressure points (see page 117), for twenty seconds each, for what's sometimes called facial 'colour-puncture'; or focus it on the points that represent chakras (see page 150).

Bright white light from a 'light box' can counteract pre-menstrual problems and seasonal affective disorder (SAD). Blue and red light from a Dermalux lamp can help acne and, perhaps, rosacea. Red flashing light from a visor (LightMask) eases pre-menstrual syndrome. And professional O-LYS coloured-light treatment is said to decrease puffiness, make skin glow, heal acne and reduce fine lines by 50–70 percent. (Details of these products are on pages 156–7).

Boost your spirits with carefully chosen colours for paints, furnishings and clothing. Red stimulates, and raises blood pressure; blue soothes, and lowers blood pressure. Your automatic choice may be what you most need for healing, or may represent a low mental and physical state – in which case you might be better off with its complementary colour.

Benefit from plant pigments by eating fruits and vegetables of many hues. And experiment with 'solarized' water – water exposed to coloured sunlight. Secure a gel of your chosen colour around a glass, or use a coloured glass or bottle. Fill with water and stand it in sunlight for one hour in summer, three to four in winter. Keep in the fridge up to three days and sip throughout the day. Avoid red solarized water in the evening as it may interfere with sleep.

cranial osteopathy

Part of your natural facelift may include visiting a cranial osteopath for treatment and, perhaps, tips on posture and movement. This therapist focuses on the skull and uses massage, plus small manipulations of the skullbones, to treat such things as depression, headaches, balance problems, ringing in the ears, sinus trouble and whiplash injuries.

Cranial osteopathy can also relieve the stress that accompanies prolonged facial pain or other symptoms. Easing stress-induced facial tension benefits the face, so preventing the development of the lines and wrinkles that are associated with abnormal tension in underlying muscles.

Cranial osteopaths believe mal-alignment of the skullbones, following an injury, for example, can impede the flow of the cerebrospinal fluid around the brain, or press on the brain, nerves or blood vessels entering and leaving it. Their gentle work satisfies many customers. But as yet no trials have been done to prove it works.

homeopathy

The name of this gentle system of medicine comes from the Greek homos (same) and pathos (suffering). It aims to boost the body's natural healing power to deal with symptoms by using tiny doses of a substance that, in a much larger amount, would cause those symptoms. So 'like cures like'.

Homeopaths believe the more dilute a remedy, the greater is its strength; their most potent remedies contain no molecules of the substance they are made from. How these could heal isn't clear. One suggestion is that a remedy's electro-magnetic frequency boosts an ill person's weakened electro-magnetic field, just as a vibrating tuning fork initiates or increases vibration in a similar, adjacent fork – a phenomenon called resonance. Another is that the molecules of the liquid in which a substance is shaken become electro-chemically charged, allowing them to 'memorize' the substance's electro-magnetic properties and aid healing

without causing the negative effects that the original substance iwould do.

Buy homeopathic remedies for skin problems, and for stress and any other conditions that indirectly affect the skin, from pharmacies and health stores. Choose the best remedy for your needs by matching your symptoms with the symptom lists in a homeopathy manual. Most remedies sold for treating symptoms are either in the 6c or 30c concentration. But a remedy is only likely to be effective, say homeopaths, if it's the right remedy, meaning it is made from a substance that would, if you took it before it was homeopathically diluted, cause the very symptoms you currently have.

If a remedy is going to work, it will probably begin to make you feel better either within a few hours or a few days. However, success from a homeopathic remedy may well begin with a 'healing crisis', in which the symptoms temporarily get worse before they get better.

Consult a homeopath about serious or long-lasting disorders. This is because in this situation homeopaths often like to recommend a person's own 'constitutional' remedy – the one made from the substance whose effects in the body are described in homeopathic tables as best matching your usual physical, mental and emotional tendencies as an individual.

sound

Sound waves are ripples of energy vibrations that travel through gases, solids and liquids from one molecule of matter to another. (This contrasts with light and other electro-magnetic rays, which are ripples or packets of energy that can travel through a vacuum.) The effects of electro-magnetic rays vary according to their wavelength. The same is true of the actions of the sound waves in the 'sound spectrum'.

Sounds vary from very high-pitched, high-frequency (short wavelength) ones, to very low-pitched and low frequency (long wavelength ones). The highest-pitched sounds are inaudible, but can still affect us in ways other than via our ears. The lowest-pitched ones are also inaudible, though we may feel some of them as rumblings or vibrations deep in our body.

Sounds have hugely important effects on body, mind and spirit. Each molecule in our body constantly vibrates, with the various tissues in the body vibrating at particular rates and intensities in health and disease. The vibrations of a sound may resonate with these intrinsic vibrations of a particular part of the body, so boosting their intensity. The theory is that this could help healing. Some eastern systems of medicine suggest that notes of different pitches affect different chakras

(see page 150) and hence the parts of the body they represent; the lowest sounds affecting the lowest chakras and vice versa.

Try out sound therapy for such things as stress, and muscle tension in your face, by:
- Listening to different types of music – high- or low-pitched, loud or soft, with varying melodies and forms – to see if any helps.
- Chanting on one note, and varying this to see which, if any, helps by patiently moving the back of your mouth and throat into different positions while chanting, you will eventually find that you can produce two notes at once; doing 'overtone chanting' is a particularly potent way of relaxing.

harnessing electricity

Many electrical devices are sold to improve the quality of the facial skin and muscle. While a healthy diet, effective stress management, massage and whole-body exercise generally do this very well, certain of these devices may add to their effects. First, however, what is electricity? Is it safe? And can you use it at home?

Electricity is a form of energy associated with static or moving electrically charged particles. Chemical reactions continuously create minute electric currents in all our cells. These currents are generated as sub-atomic particles called electrons move tiny distances from one atom or group of atoms to another. Electricity also flows when electrically chargeable atoms (such as tiny particles of iron in red blood cells) move within the body while it is in an electro-magnetic field. Such fields are all around us. The earth creates its own weak field; and power lines, both domestic and commercial, also have them, as does every item of electrical equipment connected to the mains or a battery.

Operated carelessly, any electrical appliance used on the face can cause a shock, so be sure to follow the instructions carefully.

Some electrical ('electronic' if they have more complex micro-circuitry) devices may safely improve your face's texture, circulation, fitness and firmness at home.

WHAT ELECTRICITY DOES IN YOUR SKIN

Electricity – electric power – is one of several forms of energy that affect the body. Their effects on the skin and the ways they inter-relate are fascinating.

Our body draws chemical energy (measured in calories) from food and either uses or stores it. The body stores energy from the heat around it by increasing the rate at which its molecules vibrate. It also absorbs light and other electro-magnetic (e-m) rays; takes in sound and converts it to electro-chemical energy; and benefits from external kinetic energy (the force of a moving object) from, for example, the pressure of a massage.

The body additionally produces energy from many of the chemical and electro-chemical reactions that occur during its everyday metabolism. And it experiences energy changes such as the creation of small electric currents when in the presence of an e-m field.

Some sorts of energy are interchangeable. For example, kinetic energy from a massage creates heat in the skin; so too do the e-m and electro-chemical energy of infra-red light.

In various parts of this book we touch on the physical and mental benefits obtainable from heat, light, sound, food, homeopathic remedies and massage. Devices that send an electric current into the skin also have potentially beneficial effects. An electric current applied to the skin can:

- Make it warmer, because it produces direct heat and widens arteries – which then bring more blood to the area.
- Discourage puffiness by enhancing the circulation, which increases the removal of surplus tissue fluid.
- Aid healing, by its circulation-enhancing effects and by the local stimulation of collagen and elastin production.

- Exercise muscles by altering the way their cell membranes, and those of their nerves, handle calcium, so making them contract. This is called electric (or electronic) muscle stimulation.

ELECTROMAGNETIC FIELDS

An electro-magnetic field (emf) surrounds anything powered by an alternating electric current and subjects things within it to electric and magnetic forces. We encounter emfs frequently during everyday life. So what do they do to you and your skin?

The body conducts electricity, so an emf can trigger the flow of electricity in the skin and body. The earth's emf doesn't do this because it's weak and relatively static. But many other emfs in our homes, offices and outside do.

According to scientists, extra-low-frequency (ELF) emfs can interfere with the low-frequency electrical messages used by the body's internal communication system. This could disrupt both nerve cells and the immune system's white cells. Researchers are continuing to investigate whether exposure to ELF emfs can trigger migraine, sleep problems, depression, fatigue, noises in the ear and leukaemia. If emfs do have such effects, then because any illness can induce stress, the skin and face would be indirectly affected too.

If you were to go around your home with a hand-held ELF-emf monitor, you would discover that all the mains wiring and every plugged-in or battery-operated domestic electrical appliance or device, including your mobile phone, has an emf, and that the closer you get, the more intense this is. So it makes sense to unplug unused appliances, not to sit or lie too close to a working one, and to avoid sitting by the side of a computer processor, or computer or television screen, as the emf is highest here.

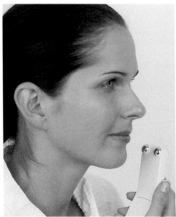

ABOVE

The hand-held battery-operated Ultratone Facial S has silver contacts that deliver a small current to the skin every two seconds. You hold it still for one minute, then move it to the next position as per the instructions.

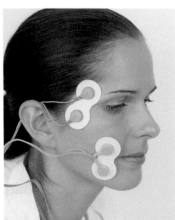

ABOVE

The battery-operated Slendertone Face has a pair of electrodes on each of four re-usable self-adhesive pads. Use two pads on each side for fifteen minutes, then move to two other positions for fifteen minutes.

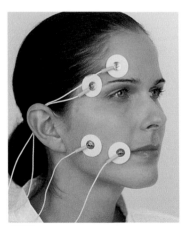

ABOVE

The CLEO II offers nine programmes and unlike the others is said to build muscle bulk. However, the nature of its eight electrodes makes it more fiddly to use than the other electronic facial stimulators.

electronic facials

The current from a facial stimulator can be delivered in one or more of many different forms. However, it is difficult for consumers to discover what, if anything, stimulators do. The market is rife with claims and counter-claims. And certain advertisements have been censured as misleading.

Electrical stimulation can brighten skin by making underlying muscle fibres contract, which boosts the local circulation. This brings more nutrients, oxygen and water to the skin, encouraging new cell growth and boosting collagen and elastin production. The stimulation pushes moisture from cream into the skin, plumping it up; but this lasts only twenty-four to twenty-eight (or, in some cases, thirty-six) hours, so must be done daily. Claims of a permanent effect led to stimulators being banned in Australia.

Heat from the increased blood flow encourages the absorption of ingredients from skin-care products and may temporarily erase fine lines by making muscle fibres contract, which stretches overlying skin. It may also temporarily erase certain lines – such as frown lines – by making already tense muscles relax.

Stimulation can make a muscle contract. However, the US Food and Drug Administration (FDA) has banned the direct sale to the public of electronic muscle stimulators marketed to help weight loss because it has seen 'no valid scientific data that these stimulators are...effective for...weight loss, shaping and contouring of the body'. In the UK there are no restrictions. So what are we to believe?

Each muscle has tens of thousands of fibres. These can be white or red, but most stimulators affect only white ones.

WHITE MUSCLE-FIBRE STIMULATION

White, (fast-twitch) fibres form only 5 percent of each facial muscle and are concentrated in its outer part. White fibres create facial expressions; prolonged use fatigues them and makes them ache.

We contract our facial muscles with everyday facial movements, but electronic stimulation – with thirty to forty pulses per second – creates an artificially large number of contractions in a short time. Such pulses are too rapid to feel, but increase the tone of white fibre, making them tighter and firmer. Repeated stimulation could 'lift' parts of the face by tightening these fibres, though because only one in twenty of a muscle's fibres are white, this would give only a very limited effect. The increased circulation brings the benefits mentioned above, reduces puffiness and shifts fat from among the muscle fibres. However, because the muscle movement is passive, it does not burn fat. The stimulation of certain facial muscles can increase expression-generated lines in the skin, so must be avoided.

INDIRECT RED MUSCLE-FIBRE STIMULATION

Red ('postural' or 'slow-twitch') fibres form 95 percent of facial muscle and make up most of its bulk. They are normally in a state of slight contraction and support the shape of the face; they do not become fatigued.

Indirect red muscle-fibre stimulation – or trophic neuromuscular (TNM) stimulation – is slow-frequency, with three to ten pulses per second, and you can feel its individual pulses. It encourages nerve endings to trigger an increase in the blood supply to red muscle fibres. This enables fibres that have become relatively inactive because of ageing to return to a higher level of contraction. TNM stimulation can therefore help prevent age-related muscle shrinkage and increases muscle bulk. This stretches the overlying skin, making it appear smoother and younger. Regular stimulation of a muscle's red muscle fibres can make it bigger.

Some facial muscles are connected to the skin. When such a muscle contracts, it squeezes this skin between its fibres. This makes skin corrugated and encourages the formation of lines. When the muscle relaxes, the skin bounces back to normal only if it's young. This is because the red fibres in ageing muscle have become less active and receive less blood. This means there is less water in them and in the attached skin. And when such a muscle relaxes, corrugations and lines are less likely to bounce back because the skin is dehydrated. However, TNM stimulation makes red fibres more active, which encourages rehydration and can help iron out lines.

ELECTRONIC FACIAL STIMULATORS

Cleo II (see page 125)

In the UK the Cleo II is the only facial stimulator available for cosmetic purposes, whose makers advocate a current causing trophic neuromuscular stimulation – the type that builds muscle bulk. This can stimulate white muscle fibres

too, but to make these bulkier, it would have to be done against some sort of resistance.

For face or body, this device comes with a waist belt. Its 'facial' chip contains a choice of programmes creating particular sequences of stimulation of various intensities and patterns. Choose from:

- general toning
- lips
- cheeks
- jaw and neck
- neck
- nose
- total eye conditioning
- eye raise
- under eyes

Ultratone Facial S (see page 125)

This hand-held, battery-operated device is the size of a mobile phone, comes in a purse and is easy to use because the electrodes don't have to be stuck to the skin. Use it for ten to twenty minutes a day.

Ultratone Futura Plus

For face or body, this comes with a waist belt. You can buy a variety of clip-in cassettes for the various parts of the body, including two for the face. Each of the facial cassettes offers four programmes, producing particular sequences of stimulation of various intensities and impulse patterns, lasting fifteen to thirty minutes each. These are:

- 'non surgical facelift' (instant lift and tone; moisture infusion; deep muscle toning; maintenance)
- 'anti-ageing facial' (fine line reduction; skin and muscle rejuvenation; rosacea treatment; lymphatic drainage).

Slendertone Face (see page 125)

This portable, battery-operated device has a neck cord and comes in a carry-case. Treating the whole face takes forty-five minutes.

part two
techniques

We have looked at the tools you need to give yourself a natural facelift: skin-care, nourishment (from within and without), face and body exercise, appropriate breathing, effective stress management, inner radiance, professional beauty secrets, massage, and certain complementary and electrotherapy techniques. Next we'll see how to use some of these to create simple yet specific techniques to help you make the various parts of your face look their best.

If you use these techniques on a regular basis, you will know that you are maximizing the way in which you present your appearance. And even if you have ever considered cosmetic surgery or other invasive cosmetic procedures, you'll know that you can now put these ideas on the back burner and have no need to take them any further.

Last but not least, using these techniques means that instead of all the fuss, bother, time, cost and risk of a facelift, eye tucks, a peel, collagen or fat implants, liposuction, jaw enhancement, nose sculpting, a brow-lift or Botox injections, you are opting for their natural alternatives. And all of these natural ways are much safer, much easier, much cheaper, much longer-lasting and, surprisingly often, just as effective as any invasive procedure – and often even more so.

YOUR EYES

putting sparkle into dull, lacklustre eyes

Fatigue dulls the eyes but is easily righted by taking measures that encourage refreshing sleep (see pages 76–7). Sometimes poor health is to blame for a lack of sparkle; if so, help boost your well-being by following the advice in Chapters 3, 4, 5 and 6, on diet, exercise, breathing and stress management.

If boredom and lack of excitement and other stimulation is wearing you down, try enriching your everyday life by adding new interests, different work and, perhaps, new relationships.

DARK RINGS, SHADOWS AND CIRCLES

Some people naturally have dark rings under their eyes. One possible reason for them is deep eye sockets, which can make this area look darker. The skin here is also relatively thin and transparent, which means its capillaries can give a bluish colour from underneath. Slower-flowing blood due to a poor circulation could accentuate this by allowing the blood to become more deoxygenated and therefore darker. Also, blood tends to pool in the skin's capillaries overnight when you are lying down in bed, making dark circles look worse in the morning. It's said that sometimes red blood cells even leak into the skin from the capillaries. The less pigment there is in the skin, the more the capillaries show, so fair-skinned people may have surprisingly dark shadows.

Sometimes dark circles result simply from melanin pigmentation; this is most likely in those with an olive or dark complexion and in fair-skinned people who've caught a lot of sun. Fatigue, poor diet, lack of exercise and dehydration may also encourage dark circles. Allergies like asthma or eczema can cause both dark rings and smooth, shiny, puffy skin.

Manage by righting any of the above causes, if possible, and by disguising the dark areas with make-up (see page 90).

In addirion, try strengthening your capillaries by:

- eating more foods rich in vitamin C and silica (leafy green vegetables, beetroot, brown rice, wholegrains, beans) and proanthocyanidins – in flavonoid plant pigments (blueberries, bilberries, other blue or black fruits)
- eating a healthy diet to foster the numbers of the bowel micro-organisms that produce most of our vitamin K
- eating bio-yoghurt each day if on antibiotics, as these kill vitamin-K-producing micro-organisms

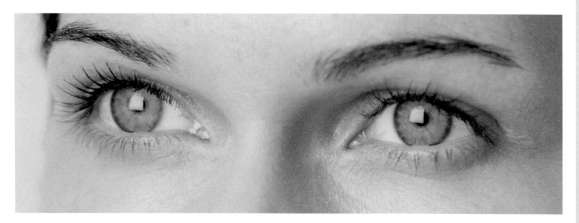

• considering supplements of proanthocyanidins and rutin, another flavonoid capillary-strengthening flavonoid.

Various eye products are marketed as being effective in decreasing dark circles. They contain such things as vitamins C or K, or proanthocyanidins. However, there is no readily available proof that they have any effect.

'GOOD' LINES OR 'BAD' LINES?

Laughter lines and crow's feet reflect the structure of bones, muscles and connective tissue; movements such as expressions and blinks; and the skin's thickness and well-being. The thin skin here is easily stretched and has few sebaceous glands. Thin skin with little oil becomes dehydrated easily – and dehydrated skin wrinkles more easily.

Smiling accentuates some lines. You can smile without moving your eyes, but most people prefer the warmth of smiling eyes. Laughter lines mark times of happiness and optimism and are generally considered as 'good' lines. Lines are accentuated by frequently narrowing the eyes (as, for example, against bright light), by smoking and by unhealthy skin.

Try these tips to minimize unwanted lines:

• Eat a skin-friendly diet and take daily exercise.

• Use good sun protection, including sunglasses.

• Stop smoking.

• Do Bates' eye exercises (see pages 134–5) and see your optician if necessary.

• Try one of the skin-care products containing retinol.

• Prescription-only 0.05 percent tretinoin cream (Retinova) is not as effective at ironing out fine wrinkles as previously thought. Also, it often causes dryness, peeling, stinging, reddening, irritation and itching. And there are persistent fears that it may damage unborn babies.

• Use (sparingly) a skin-care product containing alpha-hydroxy acids or make your own (see page 28).

• Drink enough to keep your urine pale yellow.

• Buy under-eye patches containing either collagen, glycolic acid (a fruit acid) and antioxidant vitamins A, C and E (from bioSOMME, see page 157) or plant oils and extracts (from Amirose International, see page 157); use for thirty minutes once a week or make your own.

puffy eyes

Many things can make the eyelids and surrounding skin swell. The most common is a good night's sleep! The absence of blinking during sleep allows the build-up of tissue fluid that has seeped from the capillaries. The swelling subsides as the day passes because our 10,000 or so daily blinks massage lymph vessels and capillaries, so boosting the local circulation.

Crying makes the eye area puffy, as does pre-menstrual fluid retention and too much heat or sun. Many skin creams and oily make-up removers promote overnight puffiness by leaving a greasy residue that stops the overnight surplus of tissue fluid from evaporating. Instead of these, use oil-free eye products or ones specially formulated with rapidly absorbed oils.

The thin under-eye skin is easily irritated and inflamed. The resulting swelling puts pressure on capillaries and lymph vessels so they can't carry away as much blood and tissue fluid as they otherwise would. This, in turn, causes fluid retention, which worsens the swelling. One cause is an allergy such as hay fever. Certain ingredients in cosmetics and skin-care products are also sometimes responsible, though improvements in their formulation have made this less likely. Some people are so sensitive to a particular food (such as shellfish) that their eye area swells if they even touch it after handling the food. Other causes of puffiness include eye infections, diabetes and thyroid, kidney and heart disease.

These tips may help relieve puffiness:

- Eat a healthy diet, take daily exercise and avoid smoking or passive smoking, so as to boost your circulation.
- Put a chilled, wet flannel over closed eyes for five minutes.
- Do the same with a flannel soaked in chilled green tea (available in many supermarkets and health stores), eyebright (euphrasia) or carrot tea.
- Place a cold, wet flannel over closed eyes for two minutes, then a warm one for one minute, then a cold one again, so as to boost the local circulation around the eyes.
- Rest with a chilled, wet, black or chamomile teabag on your closed eyes for five to ten minutes.
- Move an ice cube wrapped in a clean cotton handkerchief over closed eyes for a minute or two, or use a pre-chilled, gel-filled eye mask.
- Put a slice of chilled cucumber or melon over each closed eye.
- Use an eye gel containing cereal protein; this shrinks as it dries, causing temporary tightening.
- Improve the local circulation and remove excess fluid with an astringent gel containing an extract of burdock (butcher's broom) or hawthorn.
- Sleep on your back or side, with one or two pillows.
- Avoid salty foods and don't add salt to food.

EYE BAGS

Bags under the eyes result from fluid or fat. We all have fat in the skin around our eyeballs and some of us have more of this fat under our eyes than others. Ageing makes bags more noticeable because the skin becomes less elastic and the muscles lose some of their tone. This allows fat around the eyeballs to slip down and fluid and fat to stretch the skin. Changes in weight from repeated slimming also encourages bags.

Help counteract bags by:

• Identifying food sensitivities and avoiding 'culprit' foods, so as to prevent fluid retention.

• Cutting down on salt, in case it makes you retain fluid.

• Sleeping on your back, not your side, to minimize local fluid retention.

• Splashing your eyes with cold water after getting up in the morning, to reduce local fluid retention.

• Avoiding rapid weight loss or gain, to help keep skin taut.

improving your sight

Poor vision – in the form of short sight, long sight, astigmatism or ageing eyesight – plagues a large proportion of people, young, middle-aged and old. If untreated, poor vision readily makes us screw up our eyes. People do this in an attempt to improve their vision a bit, because it very slightly – and temporarily – changes the shape of the eyeballs, so altering their length from front to back.

This, in turn, allows previously unfocused rays of light (entering the eye from the thing you are looking at) to come to a more precise focus on the retina.

However, although screwing up your eyes in this way certainly may improve your vision for a few moments, doing so frequently can gradually etch permanent pronounced lines around your eyes. These include lines called crow's feet that radiate outwards from the corners of the eyes and under- and over-eye lines that curve around the eye. So clearly, if you need to improve your vision, it's wise to do this in ways other than by squinting.

Sometimes you can do nothing other than wear glasses with corrective lenses and ensure that the light is bright enough to make things as clear as possible. And remember that it's essential to visit your optician or doctor if your vision suddenly deteriorates or if you develop sudden or worsening 'flashes' (flashing lights) or 'floaters' in your field of vision.

Some people believe it is possible to improve certain eyesight problems by boosting the well-being of the various tissues in and around the eye, including the nerves, muscles, blood vessels, connective tissue and gel-like fluid that form the structures within the eyes themselves.

natural vision boosters

There are many ways in which you may be able to improve your vision.

These include:

- eating plenty of foods rich in eye-friendly nutrients: beta-carotene, vitamins A, C and E, quercetin (an antioxidant in onions and tea) and plant pigments, including proanthocyanidins (in blueberries, bilberries and other blue-black fruits) and carotenes (in red, orange and yellow fruits and vegetables): these also improve the eyes' circulation
- taking daily supplements of bilberry extract, vitamins A, C and E and quercetin
- exercising daily to improve your circulation generally
- stopping smoking – people who smoke have double the risk of poor vision in the centre of their visual field (due to degeneration of the part of the macula, part of the retina that is responsible for fine focusing)
- shielding your eyes with sunglasses in bright sunlight
- using the various techniques and exercises of the Bates method.

THE BATES METHOD

Try to improve your eyesight by using this selection of Bates techniques and exercises every day:

Splashing: In the morning splash closed eyes twenty times with warm water and twenty times with cold. In the evening splash twenty times with cold and then twenty times with warm.

Palming: Hold your palms over your closed eyes for one minute several times a day.

Sunning: Close your eyes in the sunshine and let it warm them up for half a minute or so. Gradually increase your exposure, making sure that you never get your lids burnt.

Blinking: Check that you are blinking around fifteen times a minute.

Refocusing: First, focus on something that is close up for a few seconds. Then focus on something that is far away for a few seconds. Repeat this procedure several times.

Zooming: Cover one eye and focus on a piece of paper marked with an X as you slowly bring it towards you. When the X starts to become blurred, slowly move the paper away until it is at arm's length. Repeat this procedure, gradually increasing the speed of movement.

Swinging: Hold your hand in front of you, palm down, wherever you can see it most clearly. Glance at the outer edge of your thumb, then at once glance at the outer edge of your little finger.

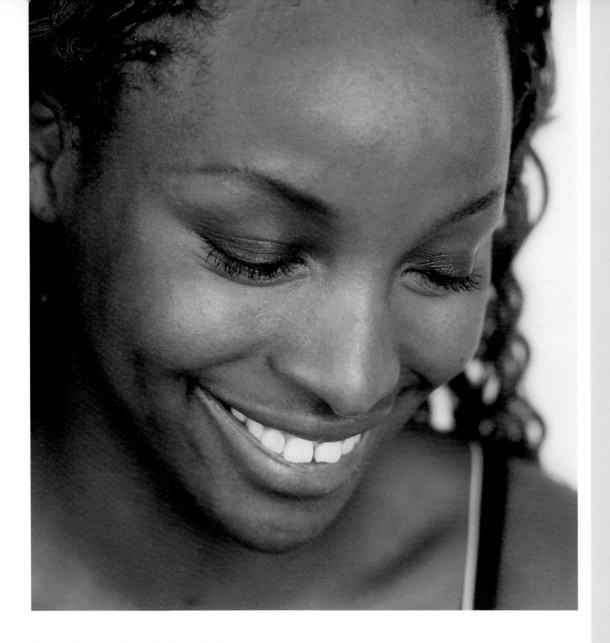

Repeat the procedure, this time swinging your
glance across only four fingers. Continue with
this process until you are glancing from side to
side of one finger.

A number of books on the Bates method explain
these and other techniques in more detail (see page
156 for some of these).

(see page 156 for some of these).

ABOVE
Check that you are blinking
around fifteen times a
minute.

YOUR CHEEKS

freckles, moles and 'age spots'

Some people consider freckles on the face beautiful, call moles 'beauty spots', and think of 'age spots' as proud badges of life's journey. Others would prefer not to have them.

Freckles are small, harmless, flat, light or dark brown marks. They contain an unusual amount of the pigment (melanin), produced by large numbers of active pigment-producing cells (melanocytes). Freckles are more common in sun-exposed skin and in very fair-skinned people, especially redheads.

Years of sun-exposure (photo-ageing) exhaust pigment cells, so melanin no longer produces an even tan but clusters in freckles. A lentigo is a pigmented mark like a light brown freckle, but is just as common on skin that is unexposed to the sun. It's often called an age freckle and is commonest in middle-aged and older people. Café au lait spots are similar but larger.

MOLES

Moles are brown, flat or raised marks and the average adult has fifteen to twenty. Freckles, lentigos, café au lait spots and moles are called pigmented naevi, though many have little pigment.

Twenty-five to forty-nine small moles on the body doubles the risk of a malignant melanoma; fifty to ninety-nine triples it.

'AGE SPOTS'

As we grow older, most of us get age spots. There are three main types: flat brown 'age freckles' (lentigos – see above); rough, yellow, brown or black, flat marks or warty growths (seborrhoeic keratoses or 'warts' – which appear stuck on and can result from sun-exposure); and red or skin-coloured lumps (solar, or actinic, keratoses – on sun-exposed skin).

So, besides triggering a build-up of melanin-producing cells, sun exposure can also lead to keratoses – lumps or patches of hard, thick skin. To help prevent or treat age spots of all sorts:

- use a sun-screening product with an SPF of 15 or more
- eat plenty of foods rich in antioxidant vitamins A, C and E, selenium and flavonoids to counter sun-damage
- try a skin cream containing alpha-hydroxy (fruit) acids
- use hydroxyquinone cream twice a day for at least six to eight weeks: this lightens age spots in six to nine people in ten by reducing melanin production
- apply a skin-care product containing retinol
- consider having a seborrhoeic keratosis removed if you dislike it
- as there is cancer risk, see a dermatologist regularly for observation of a solar keratosis or have cryotherapy treatment (freezing with liquid nitrogen), laser therapy, scraping, cutting out, cautery (heat) or chemical peeling.

Caution: If an age spot darkens, enlarges, itches or otherwise changes, see your doctor.

other blemishes

Smile lines usually enhance the cheeks but the network of fine lines that accompanies the process of ageing isn't so welcome. Scars, pigmented patches, thread veins, and the reddening of the skin known as rosacea fall into the same bracket. So just what can you do to minimize unwanted lines and blemishes?

FINE LINES AND WRINKLES

Help cheeks stay smooth and firm with the advice in Part One. Use a skin-care product containing retinol every night to treat fine lines and wrinkles. If this doesn't help after three months, ask your doctor about a prescription for 0.05 percent tretinoin cream (Retinova) but be aware that this probably isn't as effective as was first thought (see page 131). Tretinoin is a vitamin A analogue, which means it is similar to vitamin A. You apply it lightly to affected areas once daily at night until there is visible improvement, usually within three to four months, then continue applying it once or twice a week. However, researchers believe it could be absorbed through the skin in large enough amounts to damage an unborn baby, so it is unsuitable for women who are, or might become, pregnant.

Other ideas for smoothing fine lines are to splash some lukewarm comfrey tea on your face each morning to encourage new cell growth, or to apply large rejuvenating and moisturizing patches that you have either bought (for example, from Amirose or bioSOMME, see page 157) or made yourself (see pages 40–41).

SCARS

A new scar treatment helps nine out of ten raised scars and involves covering a scar with a silicone-containing gel sheet for two to four months (see *Cica-Care sheets*, page 156).

CHLOASMA (OR MELASMA)

Abnormal brown pigmentation can accompany high levels of oestrogen or other hormones that can stimulate pigment-producing cells (melanocytes). This is most likely to happen before a period, while taking the contraceptive Pill, during pregnancy or with certain thyroid, pituitary or adrenal disorders. Chloasma sometimes fades on its own and may respond to hydroxyquinone cream (see 'Age spots', page 136).

THREAD VEINS

These tiny red or blue lines, starbursts or webs are dilated capillaries. They are most common on the cheeks and nose. Causes include sun exposure, smoking, pregnancy, stress, caffeine-containing drinks, alcohol and ageing. Thread veins may accompany rosacea and can also be a sign of liver disease or a condition called lupus. To prevent or treat them:

- avoid or treat the causes, if possible
- eat foods rich in vitamin C and flavonoids
- take a supplement of vitamin C with citrus flavonoids
- try smoothing in vitamin K cream twice daily, though evidence for its efficacy is so far lacking
- smooth in twice daily for three to four weeks the contents of a vitamin E capsule mixed with two teaspoons of diluted cypress oil, one drop of neroli oil and one drop of rose, lemon or frankincense oil.

ROSACEA

The redness of rosacea results from inflammation of the skin, combined perhaps with thread veins, and is most likely in middle age. There may be pimples and, at worst, thickening and reddening of the skin of the nose. Possible causes include over-sensitivity of the blood vessels and irritation from the presence of tiny mites in the hair follicles.

Possible triggers include sunshine, temperature changes, extreme weather, stress and certain foods: spicy, fermented, pickled, marinated and smoked; liver; sirloin steak; yoghurt; sour cream; cheese, though not cottage cheese; chocolate; vanilla; soy sauce; yeast extract; dark vinegar; aubergines; avocados; spinach; citrus fruit; tomatoes; bananas; red plums; raisins; figs. Red wine and other alcohol, as well as hot or caffeinated drinks, may also be to blame.

Try one or more of these:

- Identify and avoid any triggers.
- Avoid rough flannels and towels; exfoliants; soaps; heavy hair conditioners; skin and hair products containing detergents, fragrances, oils and alcohols (found in many toners and astringents, witch hazel, hair sprays, gels and mousses).
- Use a light, non-greasy cleansing lotion, a soap-substitute or a cleansing bar or wash; moisturize afterwards.
- After swimming in chlorinated water, rinse your face by splashing with water, then moisturize well.
- Avoid using hot water on your face.
- Even when the weather is cloudy, use a non-greasy factor-15 sunscreen with UV-reflecting minerals (titanium dioxide or zinc oxide).
- Conceal redness with a light, green-toned foundation.
- Soothe with aloe vera gel or St John's wort oil (see page 115).
- Eat foods rich in vitamin B to nourish the nerves in blood-vessel walls; and in vitamin C, carotenes (red, orange and yellow vegetables and fruits) and flavonoids to strengthen blood-vessel walls (see pages 45–7 for sources).
- If hot flushes make the condition worse, eat foods rich in plant hormones (see page 47).
- Unless you suffer from a peptic ulcer, heartburn or an 'acid tummy', try taking a supplement of betaine hydrochloride – a source of acid – to improve digestion. Betaine hydrocholoride is obtainable from pharmacies.
- Manage stress more effectively.
- Massage your cheeks with featherlight strokes.
- Apply 0.75 percent metronidazole gel twice daily, or 1 percent metronidazole cream once daily.
- Isotretinoin cream (from the doctor) can help a swollen nose.
- Some people benefit from a daily session of exposure to blue and red light from a Dermalux lamp (see page 157).

RIGHT
Fine lines, acne scars, rosacea and other unwanted blemishes can be well camouflaged by clever make-up on skin of any colour.

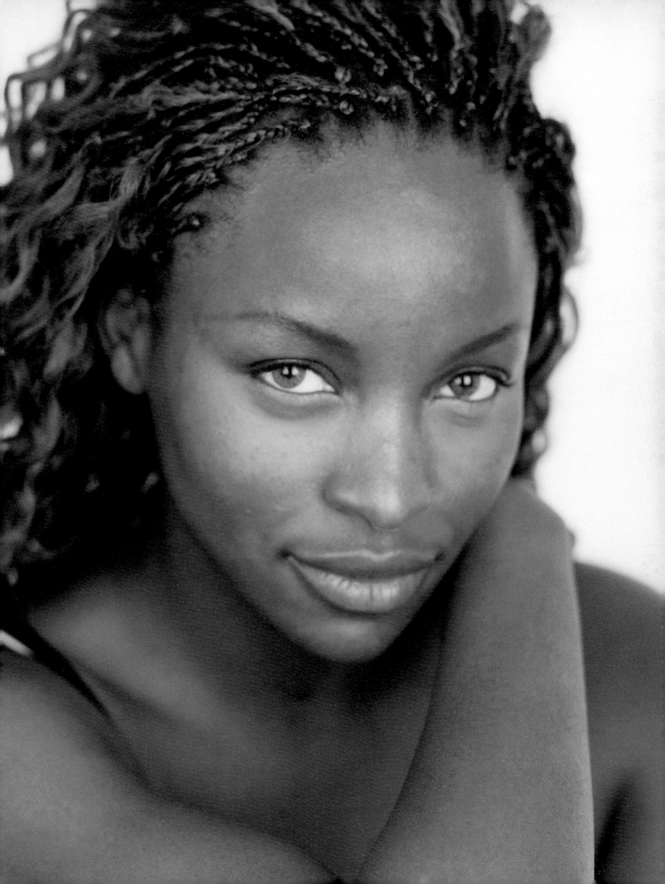

YOUR MOUTH AND LIPS

your mouth

Most people admire a generous-looking mouth with a clear shape; smooth, firm lips with unlined skin around them; and, most important, good teeth. What they don't like is a small, thin-lipped, droopy mouth with ugly teeth and little vertical lines above the upper lip.

Clearly we can't do much about the basic shape and size of our mouth without resorting to surgery. But we can enhance our looks with make-up. You can help prevent the loss of fat and colour that accompanies premature ageing. And if your reaction to the stresses of your life, combined, perhaps, with skin changes from smoking and insufficient care of teeth and gums, have made your mouth appear less than its best, there is certainly a lot you can do.

Start by boosting the health and well-being of your whole mouth area by improving your daily skin care (see Chapter 1), diet (see Chapter 3), exercise routine (see Chapter 4), breathing style (see Chapter 5) and stress management (see Chapter 6). A few other tips may help too.

SMILE

If your reaction to stress has made your mouth set in a miserable-looking expression, make yourself smile every so often. This might sound strange, but just as standing straight makes you feel better than slouching, smiling can often make you feel better than does looking unhappy. If you can make yourself laugh, so much the better.

GOOD TEETH AND A FRESH MOUTH

Some people's teeth and gums are naturally strong, attractive and healthy. Others can help prevent or treat tooth decay, gum disease or crooked, stained or missing teeth with better home care.

Tooth decay and gum disease result from acids produced by bacteria present in the mouth, as these 'eat' the remains of food left clinging to crevices around the teeth. If unremoved, bacteria-laden food traces (plaque) become hard chalky tartar (calculus), which encourages gum disease. To look after teeth and gums:

- brush your teeth on all surfaces at least once a day (or after meals) with fluoride toothpaste, and floss when necessary
- eat a mouth-friendly diet with foods rich in calcium and other minerals (to strengthen teeth) and vitamins C and E and selenium (to avoid infection and inflammation)
- clean teeth after eating foods or drinks containing added sugar, alternatively, eat some raw celery (to remove plaque), or cheese or nuts (to neutralize acid); failing this, swoosh some water around your mouth after eating something sugary
- for healthy gums, take a supplement of vitamins A, C and E and selenium, or coenzyme Q; massage gums daily to boost their circulation; and rub in aloe vera gel or rub with a fresh sage leaf to minimize inflammation.

your lips

Throughout the ages women have known that full, red, smooth lips attract men. We also like the look of them ourselves.

PLUMPING AND REDDENING LIPS

Smoothing on lipstick or lipgloss is one way of giving the mouth a blush. Another is by massaging and exercising your lips to boost their circulation and bring more blood to the surface.

Before applying make-up, massage your lips as follows:

1 Put your thumbs inside your upper lip, with your fingers outside.

2 Firmly move your thumbs in small circles. Move your thumbs and fingers to massage the whole lip. Continue for a minute.

3 Repeat with the bottom lip, this time putting your thumbs outside and fingers inside.

Exercise your lips by pursing them twenty times, or whistling for a while. Don't let little vertical lines above your top lip put you off. Boosting the local circulation makes the skin around the mouth less likely to age prematurely and settle into these lines.

The massage and exercise described above help erase these little lines or, at least, prevent them deepening too fast as you get older. This exercise is also very helpful:

1 Press the pad of your index fingertip firmly in the depression (philtrum) between your nose and upper lip.

2 Open your mouth wide, but keep your lips covering your upper teeth.

3 Smile and tighten the muscles in your upper lip for five seconds. Repeat ten times.

SMOOTHING VERTICAL LINES

If you decide to stop smoking, your circulation – and therefore the health and smoothness of your skin – will start improving as soon as two weeks after stopping.

Consider using special patches (see pages 157 for supplier) to plump up the base of each line by stimulating new cell growth. Alternatively, make your own patches (see pages 40–41).

PROTECTING YOUR LIPS

The skin of the lips is thinner than other skin, because it has only three to five layers instead of fifteen. It also has no sebaceous glands and very little protective melanin. This means it easily dries out on dry, windy, hot or sunny days and easily burns in the sun.

Protect your lips by:

• not licking them, as this eventually makes them drier

• avoiding over-exposure to the sun

• using a lipstick, lipbalm, or lipsalve with an SPF of at least 15 to protect against UV damage

• guarding against dry or windy weather with lipstick or lipbalm (see pages 37–8 for a home-made recipe) to seal in their moisture.

YOUR CHIN AND JAW

Many people admire a chin with clear, unblemished skin and with no obvious hair or a double chin. They also like the look of a clearly defined jawline. If you would like to make some improvements to the appearance of your chin and your jawline, read on.

DOUBLE CHIN

Lose excess weight, and keep it off so that your body mass index (BMI) stays within the range 20–5 (see page 50). Tone muscles with daily 'neck aerobics' exercises (see page 60).

SPOTS

The chin is a common site for spots, including both acne and the odd pimple.

Acne results from hair follicles being blocked by sticky, dead, follicle-lining cells and excess sebum (provoked by an over-sensitivity of the sebaceous glands to the hormone testosterone – which is present in women as well as men); and from infection with normal skin bacteria. Triggers include a falling oestrogen level, causing a hormone imbalance with 'testosterone dominance'; the progestogen-only contraceptive Pill; steroid drugs; the polycystic ovary syndrome; and stress. For some advice on how best to deal with acne, see page 144.

HAIR

Most 'excess' facial hair in women is within perfectly normal limits. Some women with excess hair, though, have the polycystic ovary syndrome. Other symptoms that can sometimes accompany the presence of multiple cysts on the ovaries include obesity, light or absent periods, acne, infertility and thinning head-hair. Many such women are overweight and have a history of repeated bingeing and dieting. Their condition – including their hairiness – may well improve if they lose excess weight and keep it off by eating healthily and exercising each day. A very few women have excess hair because they are taking corticosteroids (for an illness) or anabolic steroids (for body-building), or have an adrenal or pituitary problem. This can be dealt with by bleaching, shaving, sugaring or waxing. Eating more foods rich in plant hormones may help by rebalancing any hormone disruption. Professional electrolysis and laser-therapy can also be successful.

JAW-JOINT PAIN

Reduce the muscle tension and stiffness that accompany most jaw-joint pain with the advice on de-stressing in Chapter 6. Avoid draughts, relieve pain with heat (or cold if you find this more soothing), eat soft foods, massage the area and, if necessary, take painkillers. Also, see your dentist for advice; check your posture; sleep on your back with a thin pillow; and don't cradle a phone between shoulder and chin, prop hands on chin, or carry a heavy shoulderbag. Acupressure or osteopathy may help.

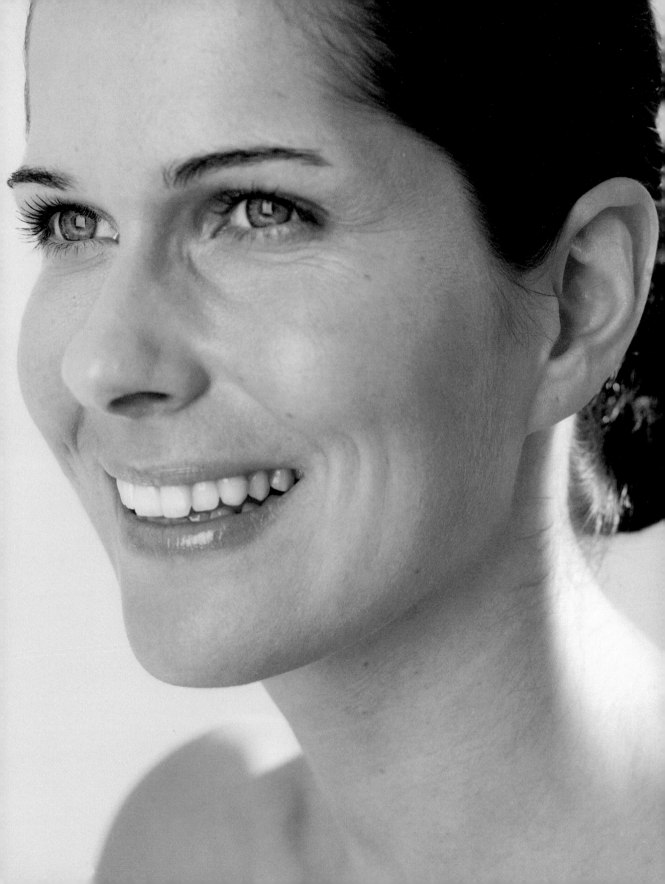

YOUR NOSE

Surprisingly many people, particularly women, wish their nose looked different. Yet you can learn to love your nose by acknowledging how important it is to your health, well-being and pleasure, and by making it look its best.

LOVE YOUR NOSE

Think positively and constructively about your nose. For example, one good thing is that it filters, warms and moistens the air you breathe. This prevents things such as flying insects, dust particles and germs from entering your throat and lungs, and stops dry, cold air over-cooling you and making your breathing passages uncomfortable. So your hardworking nose does a necessary and valuable job for you.

The other main function of the nose is, of course, to smell things. Inside its bridge is a yellowish-brown patch of fifty million 'hairs' projecting from one thousand types of odour receptor. These hairs are nerve endings, and their job is to carry smell messages to the brain that help you appreciate the flavour of food and drink. When you sip a glass of wine, for example, some of it vapourizes. Wine-laden air drifts up to the odour receptors, enabling you to appreciate the drink's bouquet.

Don't be tempted to look at your nose in isolation, perhaps wishing for a tip-tilt one when your face needs balance from the aquiline number it already has. Look at before-and-after cosmetic surgery pictures in the backs of women's magazines and you will see that some people look much better – more characterful and distinguished – with their 'birth nose'!

WHAT YOU CAN CHANGE

If you dislike your nose, define exactly what you don't like. Is it too big, long, short, wide, narrow, flared, hooked, humped or tip-tilted? Or is the texture of its skin a problem? Adjusting skin-care, hairstyle, make-up, clothing or even jewellery can make a big difference to the appearance of the nose.

SKIN CARE.

If the skin on your nose is dry and flaky, smooth in some moisturiser morning and evening. Large pores are best left alone. Contrary to what you might believe, they won't shrink with toner or any other astringent.

Deal with any acne in the following ways:

- For the occasional pimple, use oil-free skin-care products and simple patches (see page 157 and 40–41).
- Wash with facial-wash lotion or gel, or a soapless cleansing bar.
- Choose oil-free moisturizer, foundation and make-up remover lotion or gel; for oily skin, use an astringent too.
- Add a tablespoon of vinegar and two drops each of petitgrain, juniper-berry and geranium oils to 600ml (1 pint/2 1/2 cups) of water; splash your face with some of this after washing.
- Take a daily oral multi-vitamin and mineral supplement.
- Try drinking a little water containing a teaspoon of sarsaparilla (wild liquorice root or Smilax) tincture twice daily for a month.
- Eat more foods rich in plant hormones (see page 47).

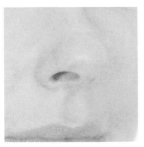 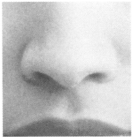 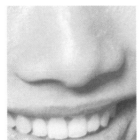 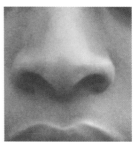

- Exercise for half an hour on at least five days a week.

- Expose your face to daylight for at least fifteen minutes each day.

- Bathe your face for fifteen minutes daily in blue and red light from a Dermalux lamp; though unproven, results seem promising.

- If you must pick a spot, wait till it points. Wash your hands, prick with a needle sterilized in boiling water or flame, squeeze gently and apply tea-tree oil.

- For blackheads, apply salicylic acid cream, gel or wash; and use a blackhead extractor or special adhesive strips.

- For persistent blackheads with greasy skin, use retinoid (a vitamin A derivative such as tretinoin, isotretinoin or adapalene) gel or lotion from your doctor.

- For persistent blackheads with dry or sensitive skin, use a retinoid or azelaic acid cream from your doctor.

- For mild acne, apply benzoyl-peroxide cream or gel, or tea tree oil. If it persists, use either some antibiotic solution, lotion or gel (used possibly alternated with retinoid cream) or some vitamin B3 cream from your doctor.

- For moderate acne, take oral antibiotics or, for women, the cyproterone acetate contraceptive Pill (Dianette), from your doctor.

- For severe acne, after two unsuccessful courses of antibiotics, your doctor may suggest oral isotretinoin.

HOW TO MAKE THE BEST OF A LARGE NOSE

A large nose can be most attractive, especially if well set off. Balance it with 'big' hair at the sides of your face, and brush any fringe back and away. Unusual or attractive earrings draw attention away, as does framing your face with a white shirt. Camouflage a high colour with concealer or foundation, and consult your doctor if you think your reddening could be caused by rosacea (see page 138) or poor circulation. If you have poor eyesight, select glasses that complement both your profile and full face, or consider contact lenses instead.

It's strange but true that some people find their nose grows in later life. This may result from poor circulation, so eat a healthy diet, exercise regularly and use effective stress-management strategies. These exercises boost the local circulation:

1 Push up your nose tip with a fingertip. Keeping the fingertip in place, attempt to bring your nose tip back down by contracting the muscle at the base of your nose. Repeat twenty times.

2 Contract and relax your nostrils. Repeat the process twenty times.

YOUR NECK AND SHOULDERS

relaxing your neck and shoulders

A stiff aching neck or shoulders can make life a misery and the resulting muscle tension can etch lines of stress deep into the skin of the face. Very often the problem stems from being unfit, lifting badly, sitting in a draught or holding one particular posture for too long – for example, when seated at a desk or driving. A less-than-comfortable bed or pillows can also be to blame, as can feeling over-stressed.

Aching is likely to be worst in the muscles above the shoulderblades (including the large, strong trapezius muscles that swathe the angle between the neck, collarbones and shoulderblades) and in the long, strap-like muscles (sternomastoids) that turn the head from side to side. If your pain continues despite home treatment, have a medical examination.

Tense trapezius muscles are often most tender where some of their fibres join the shoulderblade on each side; there may be tense bands and knots too. And you can often feel tense sternomastoid muscles as hard, tender bands down the sides of the neck.

There are several ways of reducing neck- and shoulder-muscle tension:

- If you are stressed, remember that just as mental stress encourages muscle tension (through a high adrenaline level), so having stiff muscles in turn causes mental stress. This means it's easy to find yourself in a vicious circle. Use the information in Chapter 6 to create some appropriate stress-management strategies.

- Note whether you are in the habit of tensing your trapezius muscles to lift your shoulders and ready yourself for action when you are stressed. A solution is to find a way of reminding yourself to relax them frequently. Put notes on the fridge, on your desk, in the car or anywhere, to help you do this. A second remedy is to stretch out your shoulder muscles every half-hour. And a third, if you have a sedentary job, is to invest in a chair with armrests high enough to support your elbows and forearms.

- Help prevent neck and shoulder muscles from stiffening by taking daily exercise of the aerobic, strengthening and stretching varieties (see pages 54–5).

- Eat a healthy diet with plenty of calcium- and magnesium-rich foods.

- Relax every evening by soaking in a warm bath.

- Ask your partner or another family member for a shoulder massage; alternatively, put a tennis ball on the floor, lie on your back so that the ball is beneath the tender muscles and make a small, rolling movement from side to side, allowing the ball to massage the tense muscle fibres.

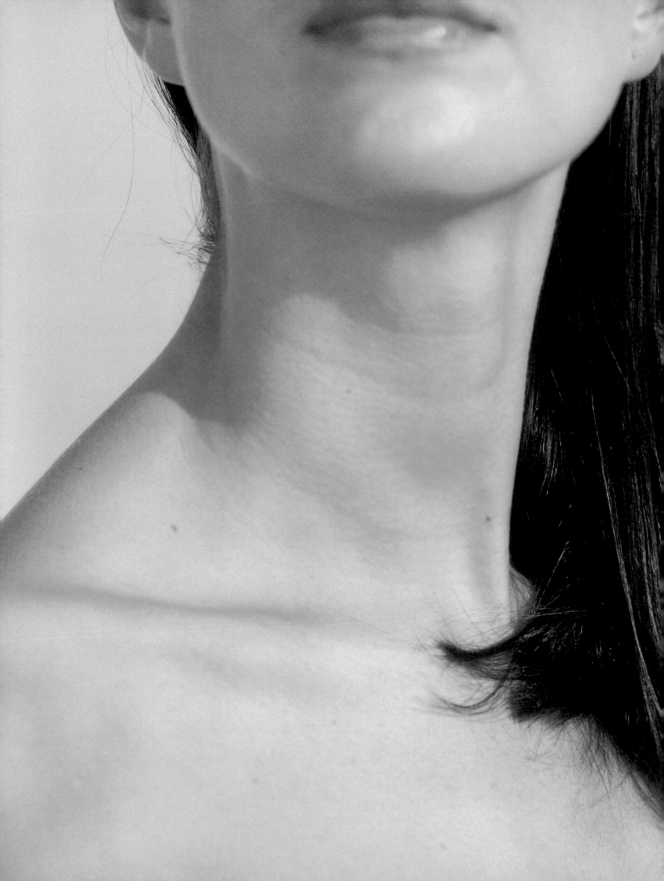

looking after your neck

The neck is exposed to the elements most of the time and is therefore very vulnerable to many daily onslaughts which affect the skin. This means we need to take extra care to protect it from UV-light exposure and the drying effects of wind and extreme temperatures.

Many people neglect this area, but there are several things you can do to prevent a prematurely aged, crêpey appearance, counteract the skin tags that are so often seen on older people, and keep your neck looking lithe, toned and slim.

SKIN CARE

Always include your neck in your usual daily skin-care routine, remembering to cleanse and moisturize it with as much 'tlc' (tender loving care) as you give to your face. And because the skin here readily dries out, use a relatively rich cream at night. Apply this after washing and patting dry, so as to seal in an extra layer of moisture. Most important, protect your neck skin from excess UV exposure by keeping it shaded when you are outside in strong daylight or using a product with an SPF of 15 or more.

Guard against dullness and skin tags by boosting the circulation to your whole body, as well as to the skin of your neck. Do this by eating a healthy diet, taking regular exercise and using effective stress-management strategies (see Chapters 3, 4, 5 and 6).

Massage not only helps guard against skin tags, but also encourages brighter skin. So give your neck a massage – or ask a friend or your partner to do it for you – once a week or so. A light tapping with the flats of your outstretched fingers all over your neck increases the blood supply to the skin and underlying tissues and is surprisingly pleasant.

Enjoy the firming, invigorating action of a cool-water splash on your face each morning on waking. Alternatively, boost the circulation in the skin of your neck by using a splash containing cypress oil (see page 36) or rosemary tea (see page 115).

NECK FIRMING

Check your posture every so often. Lift your head up to lengthen it, imagining that it is being drawn up to the ceiling by a thread attached to the highest point of the top of your head. At the same time, tuck in your chin, sit or stand up straight and be aware of the stretching sensation in your neck.

Do this careful neck-stretching exercise several times a week.

1 Warm up your neck muscles first with whole-body exercise (see pages 54–5) that makes you breathe faster and boosts your circulation.

2 Bend your neck down, then turn your head slowly and gently to one side, so you look over your shoulder.

3 Repeat the process in step 2, this time turning your head to the other side.

4 Repeat the process detailed in steps 1 through 3 three times.

Caution: always do neck exercises slowly and gently, and stop if you experience any pain, dizziness or faintness. It is normal for older people to 'hear in their head' a slight 'crunching' sound coming from the muscles and ligaments at the back of the neck.

MANAGING WEIGHT CHANGES

Loose folds of crêpey skin are an unwelcome but common result of repeated rapid weight changes. Many people in affluent developed countries frequently go on a slimming diet because they simply aren't aware of the psychological, practical and dietary skills involved in keeping to a healthy, steady weight. However, the repeated gaining and losing of excess pounds repeatedly stretches the skin as fat accumulates, then makes it sag as fat melts away again. Skin is usually remarkably efficient at accommodating changes in underlying tissues. But stretch and release it too quickly and too often, and it may not cope. Instead of remaining smooth as the underlying tissue shrinks, it then remains loose and gradually comes to hang in folds – leading to what is graphically called a 'turkey neck'.

If you need to lose weight, do it slowly, at an average of 450–900g (1–2lb) a week, particularly if you are over forty. Many people on a steady, healthy-eating weight-loss plan lose a little more during some weeks, a little less in others. Some weeks they may lose nothing or even, in the case of some women before a period, for example, put on a little temporarily; but this doesn't matter – it's the total loss over the weeks that is all-important.

SHOWERING

One wonderful therapy for the neck and, indeed, for the whole person involves standing under a shower. This stimulates the circulation in the skin and muscles of the neck and leaves you feeling relaxed and refreshed. Check the water is warm, then arrange the shower so it sprays on to the back of your bent neck, just below the base of your skull. Just stand there and note the surprisingly pleasurable tingle. Continue for as long as you like, then adjust the temperature of the water to cold and stand with the back of your neck under it again for half a minute or so. Repeat once more with a warm spray followed by a cold one.

HAIRS

Many women, especially those with certain skin types, such as dark-haired women of Mediterranean origin, have a few unwanted long, dark or coarse hairs on their neck, and some have a considerable growth. This is usually quite normal, and if you don't like it, there are several ways of dealing with it.

- Pluck the hairs with tweezers, a bright light and a mirror. This does not make them grow stronger, coarser or darker. However, it's important not to damage the skin, because repeated damage could cause discolouration or scarring,.
- Stop smoking, as this encourages facial hair.
- Bleach it.
- Have it treated with laser therapy or electrolysis.
- If you are concerned that your hairiness is abnormal, see your doctor. The most common cause of abnormal hair growth on the neck or face is the polycystic ovary syndrome (see page 142); another cause is taking corticosteroid drugs.

YOUR BROW AND SCALP

The forehead has fascinating intellectual, spiritual and mystical connotations that are surprisingly relevant to facelifts. Indeed, some of the best ways of caring for and 'lifting' the forehead are those that aid mental and physical relaxation, clarity of thought and spiritual awareness.

Behind the brow lies the brain and, according to some, the soul. The centre – where Indian women signify their married state by painting a red tika mark or sticking on a pretty decoration called a bindhi – is the seat of the 'third eye', a mystical concept representing deep, intuitive wisdom. According to oriental healing traditions, this is also the site of the sixth chakra.

THE CHAKRAS

The concept of chakras is a feature of traditional Chinese, Tibetan, Hindu, Sufi and Hopi writings. *Chakra* means 'wheel', and each chakra is conceived as a whirling vortex that transforms the frequency of energy so that it can pass between the body and the body's surrounding energy fields. The existence of a complex energy field around the body has some scientific backing. However, there is no evidence for energy-transformation centres, though the stated positions of some chakras do correspond roughly to those of certain endocrine glands. As yet chakras remain mystical entities – nonetheless they are probably useful for that.

Seven chakras are described, and these lie in a line down the front of the body:

- The first, or root (*muladhara*): in the genital area.
- The second (*svadisthana*): midway between the pubic bone and umbilicus.
- The third (*manipura*): at the solar plexus (or, for Hindus, the umbilicus).
- The fourth (*anahata*): at the heart.
- The fifth (*vishuddha*): at the base of the neck.
- The sixth (*ajna*): in the forehead.
- The seventh, or crown (*sahasranra*): in the air just above the head.

HOW CAN AN UNDERSTANDING OF CHAKRAS BENEFIT THE FACE?

The chakras are said to 'open' in turn throughout life, starting at conception, with each taking six years to open in women and seven in men. If a person's needs are being fully met, the chakra currently opening unfolds fully. If they are not, it remains partially closed, leading to less–than–optimal physical, psychological or spiritual health related to the level of that chakra.

Some alternative therapists describe their work as opening any chakras they believe to be partially closed. They do this with techniques such as breathing exercises, massage of a particular level of the body, or chanting on a note chosen for an individual chakra – the higher the chakra, the higher the note. The Indian health-care system known as *ayurveda* recommends working on the sixth chakra with a particularly relaxing therapy which they call *Shirodhara* (see pages 154–5).

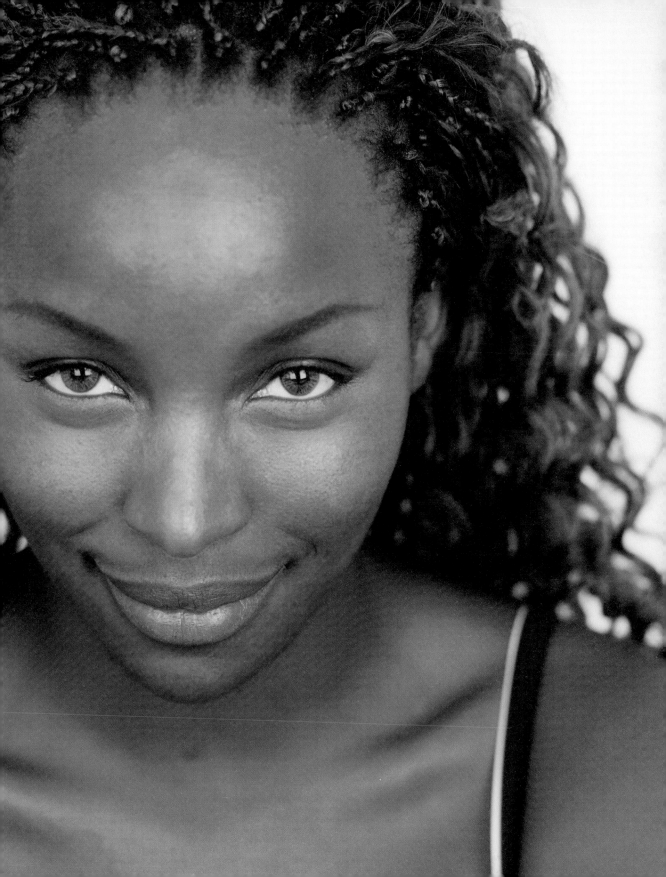

de-furrowing, patches and massage

Sometimes the habit of frowning is hard to stop simply because you forget what it is like not to frown. Relaxation exercises several times a day can help:

ANTI-FROWNING EXERCISES

Relaxing vertical lines

Close your eyes and release vertical furrows by putting your thumbtip above one eyebrow and your index fingertip above the other. Without lifting them from the skin beneath, press them apart for half a minute. At the same time release the resistance in the underlying muscles, and remember how this feels.

Relaxing horizontal lines

As for the preceding exercise, but this time putting your index fingertip at the top of your forehead and your middle fingertip at the bottom.

Once you know how it feels to have a relaxed forehead, you can repeat both these exercises any time you realize you are frowning, or think you might be.

PATCH TECHNOLOGY

If you want your forehead to look unlined for a special occasion, use patch technology. This is well researched and surprisingly successful. Buy shaped cotton-gauze patches impregnated with such things as herbal extracts and vitamins (such as Wrinkle Miracle or bioSOMME's, see page 157), or make your own (see page 41). A patch left on your lines for up to thirty to forty-five minutes moisturizes the skin so deeply that it plumps up and sheds its lines, albeit only for a day or two at most.

SCALP MASSAGE

Having a scalp massage can be blissful. You can do it yourself or have someone else do it for you. You can enjoy it while lying down, sitting in a chair or standing in the shower. And it can be done dry, with oil, or wet, with shampoo or conditioner on wet hair.

There are no rules – just do what feels best. If someone else is doing it, guide them by saying what you particularly like. The aim is to enjoy it and relax any tension in your scalp muscles. And you'll find this is most likely if you keep the massage going with continuous gentle almost wave-like movements.

1 Start by gently stroking the scalp all over with the flats of your fingers (the undersides of your stretched fingers).

2 Continue with a firm fingertip massage of the area above each ear, making small, circular movements.

3 Massage over the whole scalp with slightly bigger circles, using the flats of your palms and fingers, and taking care not to drag the hair.

4 Do long, slow strokes with the flats of your hands all over the scalp – starting each one at a different point of the hairline and moving to the crown.

5 Finish with similar strokes, but now with the fingertips. As you come to the end of each stroke, take a little bit of hair between your fingertips and slowly and gently slide them all the way from the root to the end, very very gently pulling the hair. This can feel particularly soothing when someone else does it for you.

INDIAN HEAD MASSAGE

The Indian culture offers a lovely way of looking after the scalp and hair. Indeed, the very word, 'shampoo', comes from the Indian word, champi, meaning head massage, for this is what many Indian people do to keep their scalp healthy and tension-free, and their hair clean and looking good.

A regular massage with aromatic oil is easy for a friend or relative to do for you or for you to do yourself. Some types of Indian head massage combine a popular method of scalp and hair care with the age-old methods of India's traditional health-care system, ayurveda (see page 150). This involves the belief that massaging the head influences the state of the chakras (so-called energy centres) at the levels of the crown of the head, the brow and the neck. While western science doesn't recognize chakras, we know that certain vitally important hormone-producing glands lie at the same levels. So perhaps (though this is unproven) a massage of the head (and neck) is somehow beneficial to these glands.

Although you can massage the head with bare, unoiled hands, it is even more relaxing if you choose to do it with scented oil.

Choosing the oil

According to traditional wisdom, choose the oil according to your basic ayurvedic 'type' (see page 154), or according to the seasons of the year as follows:

For spring: coconut oil (see note below)

For summer: sesame or olive oils

For autumn: almond oil

For winter: mustard oil

Ideally, warm the the bottle of oil in a bowl of warm water first; this is a must if using coconut 'oil', as this is solid at room temperature. To add a wonderful fragrance and a relaxing or stimulating dimension, add a few drops of essential oil (see pages 104-5).

Doing an Indian head massage on yourself

Put some oil between your hands and begin, using the techniques outlined for the scalp (see facing page), face (see pages 100–09) and neck (see page 148). Include the ears by gently squeezing all around the border of each one, then repeating – but this time gently pulling the border.

Doing an Indian head massage on someone else

Check the room is warm and draft-free, and use candlelight or other soft lighting. Sit the person comfortably in a straight-backed chair with their legs uncrossed, feet flat on the floor, and hands resting in their lap. Ask them to remove any ear-rings, necklaces, hairbands, or other jewellery or ornaments. Stand behind them, relax, and then follow the above guidelines. The person might also want to loosen or remove some clothing so you can massage their shoulders and upper arms too.

shirodhara

This surprisingly delightful experience involves lying with your forehead under a stream of warmed vegetable oil. It is good for relieving the muscle tension responsible for frown-lines, and with ingenuity and a friend or partner, you can enjoy it at home.

You need a rolled-up towel, a small sheet of polythene, a demi-john with a tap (as used for making wine), a photographic developing tray (or other large shallow container) and 2.3 litres (4 pints/10 cups) of suitable oil. Ayurvedic practitioners describe three basic types of people (*vata*, *pitta* and *kapha*) and suggest:

- Olive or sesame oil ('calming') for *vata* people, such as many of those who are active and have a small build.
- Sunflower oil ('cooling') for *pitta* people, such as many of those who are moderately active and have a moderate build.
- Corn, safflower or sesame oil ('burning') for *kapha* people, such as many of those who are slow and have a large build.

You can scent the oil used with ten drops of lavender oil.

2 Warm the oil to just above body heat, pour into the demi-john and put this on a table so that the tap clears the edge.

3 Lie on the floor with your forehead under the tap and the towel under your neck. Tuck one edge of the polythene sheet under your head, bring the tray up to your head and put the free edge of the sheet into it so it catches the oil from your forehead.

4 Now you can relax while your friend turns on a thin stream of oil.

5 When it is finished, your friend can use some of the oil to give you a slow, relaxing scalp massage.

SPOTS

Acne (see pages 144-5) favours the forehead because this has so many sebaceous glands. Other culprits include fringes ('bangs') and hairstyling products such as firm-hold hair spray that can block follicles or irritate skin. Consider shorter hair or a swept-back hairstyle, and protect your forehead when applying styling products.

FROWN-LINES

Tensing the forehead's horizontal or vertical muscles creates corrugations at right angles to the muscles themselves. Some people furrow their brow when stressed or concentrating, others when straining to see or protecting their eyes from the wind or a bright light. And some frown from displeasure or disapproval.

You develop a permanent furrow if you frown at least 200,000 times. To prevent this or to reduce existing lines, discover the triggers that make you frown. You may then need to:

- Find better ways of reacting to stress (see Chapter 6) that do not include frowning.
- Improve your vision with glasses or Bates exercises (see pages 134–5). These exercises include splashing your closed eyes with cool water; looking into the distance

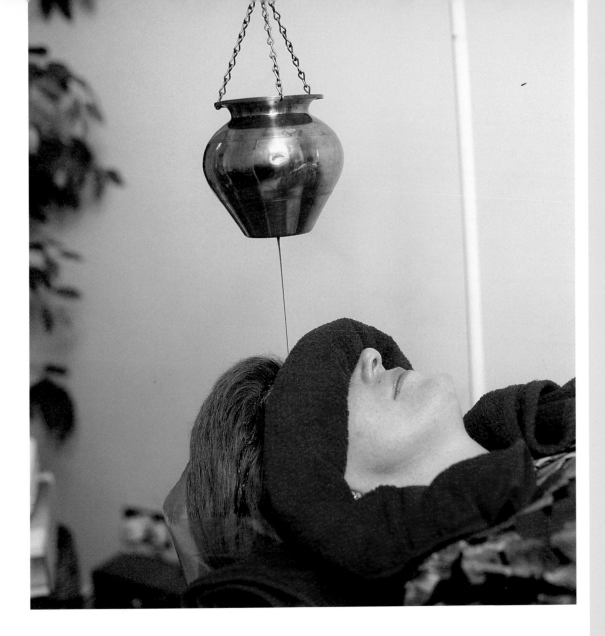

frequently when doing close work; and 'palming' –
covering your eyes with the palms and relaxing.

- If you have dyslexia and frown when reading words that
appear to be jiggling around, visit an optometrist with a
colorimeter (see Cerium Visual Technologies, page 156).
Lenses of a precisely chosen tint may help 'keep words still'.

- Protect your eyes from bright light and high wind.

- Get your partner, a member of your family or a close friend

to tell you when you are frowning. It's all too easy for it to
become an unconscious habit. But it's one that with
patience and persistence you can readily be broken.

- Use Anti-Wrinkle Collagen Patches (see page 157 for supplier).
Their collagen, glycolic acid and vitamins A, C and E stimulate
cell growth in the base of each furrow; one application is said
to reduce lines by 60 percent and benefits are cumulative.
Alternatively, make your own patches (see pages 40–41).

HELP LIST

books

Buenaventura, Wendy, *Beauty and the East* (Saqi Books, 1997)

Busch, Julia, *Treat Your Face Like a Salad* (Anti-Aging Press, PO Box 141489, Coral Gables, Florida 33114, 1993).

Gibson,Dr H. B., *A Little of What You Fancy Does You Good* (Third Age Press, 1997).

Hampton, Aubrey, *Natural Organic Hair and Skin Care* (Organica Press, 4419 N. Manhatten Avenue, Tampa, Florida, 1990).

Liberman, Jacob, OD, PhD, *Light – Medicine of the Future* (Bear & Co, 1991).

Loughran, Joni, *Natural Skin Care* (Frog Ltd, c/o North Atlantic Books, PO Box 12327, Berkeley, California 94712, 1999).

Lowe, Professo, Nicholas MD and Sellar, Polly, *Skin Secrets – the Medical Facts versus the Beauty Fiction* (Collins & Brown, 1999).

McIntyre, Anne, *Complete Floral Healer* (Gaia Books, 1996)

Mackie, Rona M, *Healthy Skin – The Facts* (Oxford University Press, 1992)

Mansfield, Peter, *The Bates Method: A Complete Guide to Improving Eyesight Naturally* (Trafalgar Square, 1997).

Roth, Gereen, *Breaking Free from Compulsive Eating* (Plume Books, 1993)

Stanway, Penny, *Healing Foods for Common Ailments* (Gaia Books, 1995); *Natural Well Woman* (Element, July 2000)

Weeks, Dr David and James, Jamie, *Superyoung* (Hodder & Stoughton, 1998).

suppliers

Many companies can mail worldwide.

UK

Aqua Oleum – essential and carrier oils;
(00 44) 1453 753555.

Bach Flower Remedies – flower remedies;
(00 44) 1235 550086.

Cerium Visual Technologies – a list of optometrists with a colorimeter from (0044) 1580 765211.

Cica-Care sheets – for scars, from some pharmacies; each piece used must be cleaned twice daily and replaced withinin a month; (00 44) 1482 673 508.

Cleo II – electrical facial stimulator, from the Kaymar Group Ltd; (00 44) 113 2527744.

Colour Me Beautiful – colour-choice consultations;

(00 44) 207 627 5211.

Dermalux – a lamp producing blue and red light used for acne and rosacea; details from the UK manufacturer on:

(00 44) 800 0722122.

LightMask – for pre-menstrual syndrome;

(00 44) 980 168143.

Patches for pimples – with herbal extracts, kaolin and salicylic and lactic acids, from Amirose International (see Wrinkle Miracle below).

Potter's Herbal Supplies Ltd – herbal supplies;

(00 44) 1942 234761.

Quitline – stop-smoking information;

(00 44) 800 00 22 00.

SAD Light Box Co. – light boxes for light-deficiency depression; (00 44) 1494 448727.

Slendertone – Face (electronic facial stimulator) from Slendertone UK; (00 44) 345 697 278.

Ultratone – (electronic facial stimulator) from Ultratone Bodyshapers; (00 44) 207 935 0631.

Vitamin K creams – derm-A-Klear, M.D, a cream containing vitamin A, 1 per cent vitamin K, and aloe vera, from UK Home Shopping on (0044) 800 698 7541; and Dermal-K, with 5 per cent vitamin K, from

(00 44) 208 208 0616.

Wrinkle Miracle – shaped cotton patches impregnated with a selection of the following: avocado, wheatgerm, jojoba, camomile, sage and sweet-almond oils; fenugreek; and beeswax. Sold in separate packs for under eyes, between eyebrows, for cheeks, upper lips, neck or forehead; from Amirose International on

(00 44) 208 554 3335.

USA

bioSOMME's Anti-Wrinkle Collagen Patches – contoured patches containing collagen, glycolic acid and vitamins A, C and E, sold in separate packs for under eyes, upper lips or forehead from 1 800 591 1667.

Capitol Drugs, Inc. – nutritional supplements, and herbal and flower remedies; 1 800 858 8833.

Simpler's Botanicals – essential oils and carrier oils; 1 800 652 7646.

AUSTRALIA AND NEW ZEALAND

Martin & Pleasance Pty Ltd – flower remedies from PO Box 2054, Richmond, Vic. 3121; (03) 427 7422.

Vitamin Supplies Pty Ltd – vitamins and other health supplements from 51–55 Warrah Street, East Chatswood, Sydney, NSW.

websites

Dermalux (see above) – at www.dermalux.co.uk.

Cleo II – electrical facial stimulator, at www.kaymargroup.com.

Herbal remedies – a commercial site with information about herbs, on-line ordering and an e-mail Q and A service at www.allherb.com.

National Sports Medicine Institute of the UK – exercise and fitness tips at www.nsmi.org.uk.

O-LYS Light Treatment – www.o-lys.com.

Quit – stop-smoking information at www.lifesaver.co.uk.

Slendertone – Face (electronic facial stimulator) at www.slendertone.co.uk.

index